FUR-EVER FRIENDS:

A Journey with Your Sacred Companion

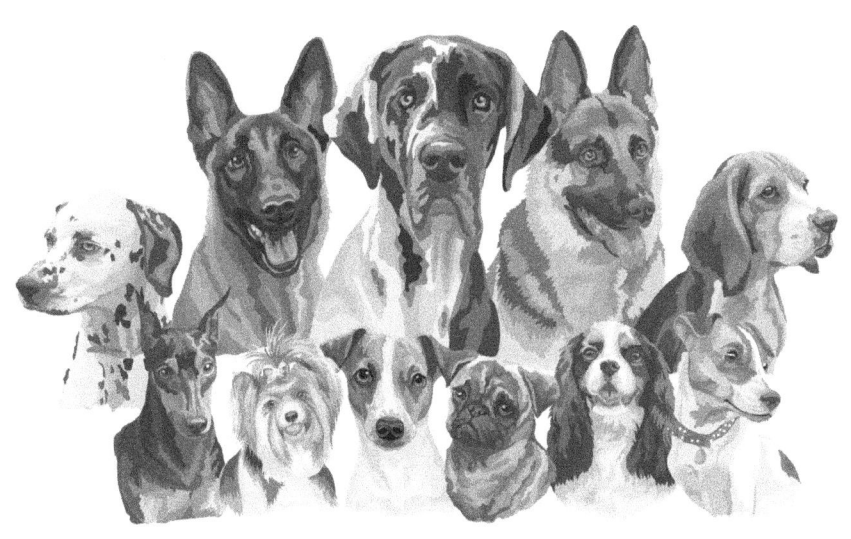

Sean James

Fur-Ever Friends: A Journey with Your Sacred Companion

Copyright © 2025 by Sean James
Los Angeles, California
fureverblessed2025@gmail.com
All rights reserved.

Printed and bound in the United States of America

Published by Cole Publishing

No reproduction of any part of this format, contents or artistic contributions can be made without written permission from the author.

Library of Congress
Cataloging-in-Publication Data
ISBN: 979-8-9918058-8-9

Cole Publishing
4067 Hardwick Street #282
Lakewood, CA 90712

Email: Colepublishing2000@gmail.com
Book Cover Design by Cole Publishing

For Book Orders:
Contact us at Cole Publishing Company
www.ColePublishing.org

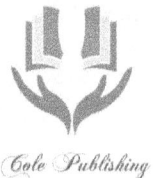

CONTENTS

DEDICATION V

ACKNOWLEDGMENTS VII

PREFACE IX

INTRODUCTION XIII

CHAPTER I:
A Gift from God 19

CHAPTER II:
Love Without Words 51

CHAPTER III:
Companionship in Every Season 65

CHAPTER IV:
Lessons from [Your Dog's Name] 79

CHAPTER V:
A Reflection of God's Love 99

CHAPTER VI:
Gratitude for the Journey 111

CHAPTER VII:
A Prayer for You and [Your Dog's Name] 129

CHAPTER VIII:
The Power of Your Words 149

THANK YOU 167

SCRIPTURAL REFERENCES 169

REFERENCES 173

ABOUT SEAN JAMES 175

DEDICATION

To my friends with cherished furry companions:

To those often overlooked for not having human children but who find love, companionship, and joy in the incredible gift of animals.

To those who treasure the solace provided by their furry friends, even when society fails to acknowledge the depth of that connection.

To the individuals who leave the TV on for their pets to combat loneliness.

To those who brave inclement weather for walks, prioritizing their furry friend's happiness over their own comfort.

To those who rush to the veterinarian without a second thought, regardless of expense, because their pet's well-being is paramount.

To the caregivers who spend sleepless nights with a sick pet, whispering gentle reassurances that all will be well.

To those who purchase strollers and backpacks to keep their furry companions close, finding joy and peace in their presence.

To the travelers who willingly buy extra tickets to include their beloved companions in their adventures.

To those whose hearts have been wounded by people yet healed by the steadfast love of an animal.

To the souls who have discovered a bond that fills the void left by human relationships, offering more than they ever anticipated.

And to the Creator and King of all, the One who made us and these extraordinary creatures, who blesses us with their presence and sustains us, even in our shortcomings.

He is the Giver of all good gifts, including the privilege of sharing our lives with a furry friend.

— FUR-EVER FRIENDS —

I also dedicate this book to my mother, Christine Johnson, Star, Grace (her dogs), and my dad, Dr. Terrence A. James, for their support, assistance, and life. Thanks for everything, both of you. Love Always.

ACKNOWLEDGMENTS

I give glory to God, the Giver of life and Creator of all. Without His breath and grace, I am nothing. Everything I am and am becoming is because of Him. Thank You, Lord, for my creativity, my ability to create stories and encouraging others. This book reflects Your goodness.

I also honor three wise Kingdom men who live out their God-given purpose. Their teachings and mentorship have impacted my life and opened my eyes to the Kingdom of God.

Dr. Myles Munroe introduced me to Kingdom principles and powerful business truths from the Bible. He had a unique gift for simplifying the Word of God, making it practical and applicable. His teachings instilled in me a deep desire to study the Bible, seek God's Kingdom, and live abundantly by following His principles for success. Dr. Munroe, your legacy continues to inspire, and I am grateful for the foundation you laid in my journey.

Dr. Myron Golden enhanced my understanding of the Kingdom of God and success principles. His teaching connects God's Word to life, business, and personal growth, proving transformation. Through his YouTube channel, he empowers others by demonstrating how obedience to Kingdom principles leads to a purposeful, abundant life. Thank you, Dr. Golden, for showing me how to apply these truths in every area of my life.

Bishop Wayne Malcolm is a visionary who inspires others to fulfill their God-given purpose. He emphasizes claiming territory for the Kingdom and using our gifts in the marketplace to impact the world. His teachings have helped cultivate my abilities, align them with Kingdom principles, and share them for God's glory.

I thank these three Kingdom men for their wisdom, mentorship, and commitment to sharing Kingdom principles. Their dedication to God's Word and their zeal for helping others discover their purpose have motivated me to pursue my calling with bold confidence. I thank God for these men, their faithfulness to their missions, and the lives they have influenced, especially mine.

"I want to express my heartfelt thanks to the entire Cole Publishing family for your guidance, expertise, and unwavering patience as I started this journey as a first-time writer and author. The impact you've had on helping me bring this God-given project to life is truly remarkable. My gratitude knows no bounds.

Cole Publishing, you're a shining example of Philippians 4:19: "And my God shall supply all your need according to His riches in glory by Christ Jesus." Through your kindness, wisdom, and support, God has provided exactly what I needed during this time. From the bottom of my heart, thank you."

With a heart full of gratitude,

Sean

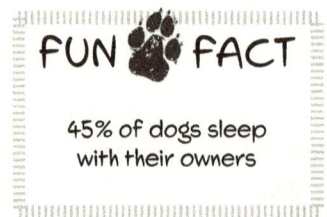

PREFACE

This book is crafted to help you recognize your dog as not merely a pet but as a precious gift from God. It provides an opportunity to reflect on your bond, document memories that highlight God's kindness, and celebrate the joy your dog brings into your life. As you write, pray, and contemplate, I hope you will view your dog as part of God's plan to love and care for you.

God's commitment to us knows no bounds. He employs everything, including people, creation, and even animals, to fulfill His purpose in our lives. Your dog is a living testament to that commitment, a visible and tangible reminder of His faithfulness and provision.

Take a moment to express your gratitude. Thank Him for the wagging tails, the sloppy kisses, the comforting cuddles, and the endless joy your dog provides. Let this book remind you that in every wag of their tail, playful bark, and quiet gaze, you are cherished by your dog and the Creator who entrusted them to you.

May this book help you develop a deeper sense of gratitude for your dog and for the God who chose to bless your life with their companionship.

With love and encouragement,

Sean

Scriptural Reminder: *"Every good and perfect gift is from above" (James 1:17).*

Your dog is one of those gifts. Celebrate them!

— FUR-EVER FRIENDS —

TAKE A MOMENT TO PERSONALIZE YOUR JOURNEY

Pause now as we begin to answer these questions over the following 2-3 pages. Feel free to use your creativity and add more engaging questions as well!

What is your dog's name, and how did you develop that name for them?

When was your dog born, or did they become part of your family? You may want to note their birth or adoption date.

What are some of your favorite memories with your dog so far?

Take a moment to write down those cherished moments that bring you happiness. I encourage you to include any drawings, photos, or illustrations in this section.

This marks the start of our adventure, so let's kick things off by having fun designing our blueprint!

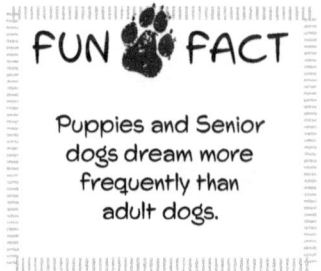

FUN FACT

Puppies and Senior dogs dream more frequently than adult dogs.

JOURNAL NOTES

— FUR-EVER FRIENDS —

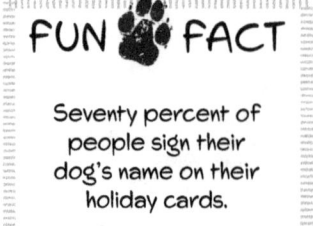

FUN FACT

Seventy percent of people sign their dog's name on their holiday cards.

INTRODUCTION

Dear (Your name here) and (Your dog's name),

Have you ever looked into your dog's eyes and felt overwhelming gratitude? That is no accident. God created animals in His infinite wisdom and love to reflect His care for us. This book is more than a journal; it is an invitation to embark on a journey of discovering the depth of God's love and provision, which is beautifully revealed through your relationship with your dog.

The Bible reminds us, **"Every good and perfect gift is from above"** (James 1:17). Your dog is one of those precious gifts, a unique blessing chosen just for you. God's love is so vast and personal that He uses His creation, including animals, to bring us joy, companionship, and even profound lessons about His character.

Think about the times your dog has brightened your day with a wagging tail, or comforted you during a quiet moment with their gentle presence. These moments are not mere coincidences but glimpses of God's goodness and intricate plan for your life.

HE IS ALWAYS WORKING ON OUR BEHALF!

A close friend who works in a hospital in a large city recently shared a powerful story with me. It illustrates how God can use our pets to bless, help, and even save us.

One night, during a particularly quiet shift in the ER, a patient was rushed in with a gunshot wound. He was a man in his 30s or 40s, and from the moment he arrived, his demeanor was prideful and sharp-witted. His life had been marked by incredible trauma, yet he had managed to overcome these challenges to achieve remarkable academic success. After obtaining a bachelor's and master's degree, he was on the verge of completing his Ph.D.

Despite his achievements, the patient dismissed those he deemed less intelligent than himself. If others were not "on his level," he would not give them the time of day. To him, most people were beneath his attention.

As he waited to be seen, a therapist entered the room. Before meeting him, she had reviewed his file, which was extensively filled with accounts of trauma, tragedy, and abandonment. Despite these hardships, his file revealed the strength and determination propelling him to his success. However, it also hinted at deep pain and unresolved struggles.

The therapist understood that this would not be an easy conversation. Although she knew the patient's attitude might be challenging, her passion for helping people outweighed any hesitations. So, she stepped into the room.

The patient greeted her with a mix of arrogance and indifference. He immediately launched into an elaborate explanation of how he had been cleaning his gun when it accidentally discharged, causing his wound. He emphasized his academic achievements, almost as if they should exempt him from being questioned.

"I'm about to receive my Ph.D.," he said. "I don't understand why everyone is treating me like some common criminal or lunatic." He went on at length, making it clear he felt the therapist's presence was unnecessary and a waste of his time. Yet, the therapist remained patient, listening carefully and allowing him to express everything he needed. When he finally paused, she responded calmly.

"I've read your file," she began. "I know about your past, the hardships you've endured, and the incredible strength it's taken to get where you are today."

As she stood to leave, she stopped and turned back to him. "I noticed you have a dog," she said, her tone shifting to one of both compassion and directness.

"I don't believe the gunshot wound was an accident. I think you intended to take your own life. But your dog, your incredible dog, saw what you were about to do and intervened. That's why you're here alive. Your dog saved you."

She began to leave the room, but the young man broke down in tears before she reached the door. Through his sobs, he admitted that everything she had said was true. Overwhelmed, he began to pour out his heart.

The therapist returned to her seat, giving him the needed space. He spoke about his dog and the joy and comfort it brought into his life. He shared the pain he had endured, the family and friends who had let him down, and how, through it all, his dog had been the one constant.

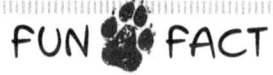

FUN FACT

Dogs can detect heat and thermal radiation, which explains how blind or deaf dogs can still hunt.

"This dog has been my anchor," he said. "My companion. My saving grace. I don't know what I would do without him."

This story reminds us of the incredible ways God works through our furry companion. They are more than just pets; they are gifts from God, sent to bring love, comfort, and sometimes even salvation into our lives. For this young man, his dog was not just a companion but a divine intervention, a reminder that even in our darkest moments, we are never truly alone.

A LOVE LETTER STORY TO [YOUR DOG'S NAME]

Oh, [Your Dog's Name], you make this house a home. With your wagging tail and cheerful roam.

When we take a walk, step by step, side by side,

I'm so thankful for you, my joy, my pride

Psalm 145:9 – "The Lord is good to all; he has compassion on all he has made."

You sit so sweetly when I say, "Good doggie!"

You're more than a pet; you're my blessing indeed.

I look at you and know God had a plan,

To place you in my life, oh, how grand!

Jeremiah 29:11 – "For I know the plans I have for you," declares the Lord.

When I say "no biting," you tilt your head.

But with a toy, you're playful instead.

Your favorite treat makes your eyes shine bright,

Oh, [Your Dog's Name], you delightfully fill my heart!

A blanket for naps, your spot on the bed,

You jump with joy when it's time to be fed.

Food in your bowl and water just right,

I thank God for you every day and night.

Psalm 36:6 – "You, Lord, preserve both people and animals."

FUR-EVER FRIENDS

Through the good days and bad, you're my dear friend,

With you by my side, my heart starts to mend.

You sit when I ask; you heal my soul, too, I'm so grateful for you, [Your Dog's Name].

When you're a good doggie, my smile beams wide,

Even when you're a rascal, I'm still on your side.

Because love is forever steadfast and true,

I'll never leave, just like God promised you.

Joshua 1:5 – "I will never leave you nor forsake you."

We walk through the seasons, rain, shine, or snow,

With you, [Your Dog's Name], my love continues to grow.

Your wagging tail tells me you're glad I'm near,

As I softly whisper, "I love you, my dear."

If you're hungry, I'm here to provide.

With a toy or a treat, I'll be by your side.

Oh, [Your Dog's Name], God made you just right,
To be my companion, my comfort, my light.

"The righteous care for their animals," it's true,

And every day, I'll take care of you.

Together we'll journey, together we'll play,

I'm grateful to God for His gift every day.

Proverbs 12:10 – "The righteous care for the needs of their animals."

[Your Dog's Name], you're more than a pet to me,
You're a gift from above, my family.

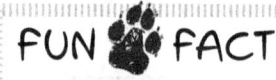

FUN FACT

When humans yawn, dogs are likely to yawn too, especially if they recognize the person.

When sleeping, dogs curl into a ball to shield their organs; this instinct stems from their wild days when they were susceptible to predator attacks.

With paws on my lap and your head on my knee, You remind me of God's love so faithfully.

So, let's jump and wag and run all around,

Let's bark with joy at the love we've found.

You're my good doggie, my little delight,

You make every day so wonderfully bright.

Oh, [Your Dog's Name], you're a blessing, it's true,

And every moment, I'm thankful for you.

So, let's end with this as I scratch your ear:

"I love you, [Your Dog's Name], my heart is clear."

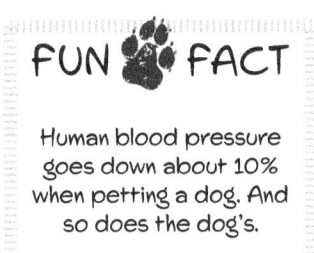

FUN FACT

Human blood pressure goes down about 10% when petting a dog. And so does the dog's.

Dear friend, God has blessed you with [Your Dog's Name], an amazing friend and furry companion. Show gratitude for the joy and companionship they bring into your life. Let this book remind you of the love between you and your beloved dog, a precious gift from our compassionate Creator.

GOD'S DEDICATION TO US THROUGH ANIMALS

Throughout history, God has used animals to accomplish His purposes to save, bless, warn, and even protect His people. Think of the ravens that fed Elijah in the wilderness (**1 Kings 17:4-6**) or the donkey that spoke to Balaam, warning him of danger ahead (**Numbers 22:21-33**). Consider Noah's ark, where God saved humanity and animals, demonstrating His care for all creation (**Genesis 7:1-16**).

Your dog is part of this story, uniquely reflecting God's provision and care. Just as God provided these animals in the Bible, He has provided your dog for you. Perhaps your dog entered your life during a season of loneliness, bringing joy through their playful antics. Or maybe they can sense when you are upset, gently resting their head on your lap as if to say, "I'm here for you."

Have you ever thought about the care God took in creating your dog? Every wag of their tail, every playful bark, and every quiet cuddle is a testament to His thoughtfulness and creativity. Your dog was designed to reflect God's love for you in a profoundly personal way.

Examples of God Working Through Your Dog

1. A Protector and Comforter

Have you noticed how your dog can sense when you are feeling anxious or upset? [Your Dog's Name] stays close by, offering comfort without needing words. This is a beautiful reminder of God's peace, which wraps around you through your dog's loving presence.

2. A Daily Reminder of Joy

After a long day, your dog eagerly greets you, wagging their tail excitedly. They reflect God's delight in you and His boundless love.

Just as your dog longs to be near you, God also yearns for you to draw closer to Him.

3. A Teacher of Unconditional Love

Your dog loves you unconditionally, regardless of your mistakes or flaws. This love mirrors God's agape love, which is limitless, unwavering, and always faithful.

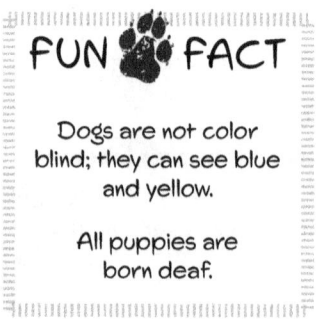

FUN FACT

Dogs are not color blind; they can see blue and yellow.

All puppies are born deaf.

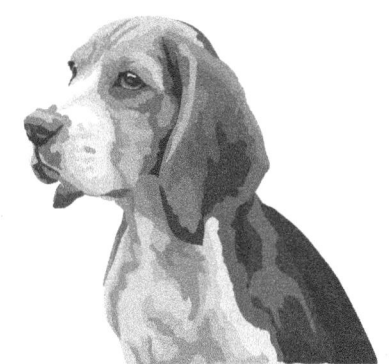

CHAPTER 1:
A Gift from God

Psalm 36:6 – "You, Lord, preserve both people and animals."

THE HEALING POWER OF GOD'S GIFT

Psalm 34:18 – "The Lord is close to the brokenhearted and saves those who are crushed in spirit."

Dogs possess an extraordinary talent for detecting our emotions. They sense when we are sad, anxious, or down, and their responses often offer solace in ways that words fail to achieve. This is not mere coincidence; it reflects God's design and His love for us.

As silent healers, dogs provide their presence as a source of comfort and tranquility. Just as God vows to be near the brokenhearted, He often utilizes His creations, like our dogs, to remind us that we are not alone. In moments when words escape us and life feels daunting, our dogs serve as tangible manifestations of God's love and care

EXAMPLES OF GOD'S HEALING IN OUR LIVES

God's Healing Through Dogs

Imagine coming home after a hard day, feeling overwhelmed. Then, there's [Your Dog's Name], wagging their tail and looking at you with unconditional love. They climb into your lap, nuzzle your hand, or lay quietly by your feet. Their presence feels like a balm for your soul, a reminder that you are loved and valued.

How God Applies this to Us

Just as your dog instinctively senses your pain and draws close to you, God draws near when we are hurting. He does not always fix the problem immediately, but His presence brings peace. Much like the comfort your dog offers, God's love surrounds us, reminding us that we are never alone in our struggles.

Reflection: Think about when your dog comforted you when no one else could. How did that reflect God's care for you?

God's Healing in Times of Grief

When we lose someone we love, the pain can feel unbearable. Many people share stories of how their dogs stayed close to them during times of grief, lying by their side as if to say, "I'm here for you." Their quiet presence can provide comfort when human words fall short.

God's presence is even more profound in our grief. He doesn't shy away from our pain, but steps into it with us. He listens to our cries, understands our sorrow, and sends us reminders of His love, whether through the people or animals He places in our lives.

Reflection: How does your dog's loyalty during your most vulnerable moments mirror God's promise to never leave or forsake you (Deuteronomy 31:6)?

HOW YOUR DOG TEACHES YOU ABOUT GOD'S HEALING PRESENCE

- Unspoken Comfort: Dogs don't need words to provide comfort. Similarly, God often speaks to us in silence through the stillness of His presence.

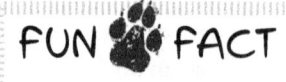

FUN FACT

Seeing Eye Dogs are trained to do their business on command, making it easier for their owners to clean up. Popular commands include "get busy" and "go time."

Petting a dog and gazing into their eyes releases oxytocin, the "love hormone," for both of you.

- Nonjudgmental Love: Dogs don't care about your mistakes or flaws; they love you unconditionally. This reflects God's agape love, which is constant and healing.
- Faithful Companionship: A dog's unwavering loyalty reminds us of God's faithfulness. They stay close, just as God promises to be near to the brokenhearted

"Healing Moments Reflection"

- Sit in a quiet space with [Your Dog's Name]. Reflect on a time they comforted you without needing to say a word.
- Write down what they did, whether it was lying beside you, licking your hand, or simply being present.
- Next, reflect on how God has comforted you in similar moments. Write down a prayer of thanks for both God's presence and the gift of [Your Dog's Name].

THE GIFTS OF GRACE AND MERCY

Like the best of friends, grace and mercy know when to speak, when to step in, and when to simply walk with you.

Grace is receiving a gift or blessing that you don't deserve.

> Biblical Example:
>
> *God gives us eternal life through Jesus, even though we can't earn it (Ephesians 2:8-9).*

Mercy is not receiving a punishment or consequence that you do deserve.

> Biblical Example:
>
> *God forgives our sins and withholds judgment because of His love (Lamentations 3:22).*

Think of grace and mercy as two sides of the same coin, both flowing from God's love: Grace gives us what we don't deserve (a gift). Mercy withholds what we do deserve (a consequence). They work together beautifully. If you break a rule, mercy is your parent deciding not to punish you, while grace is taking you out for ice cream!

Grace and Mercy in Your Relationship with Your Dog

Grace:

Your dog doesn't have to "earn" your love. You give it freely just because they are yours. Your generosity mirrors God's grace, whether it is through snuggles, treats, or playtime.

> Example: Think of a time when your dog accidentally knocked something over or made a mess, but instead of scolding them, you gave them a treat because you couldn't resist their cute face. That's grace: receiving a blessing when it was not earned.

Mercy:

Dogs can get into trouble chewing on shoes, digging in the yard, or barking at everything. Instead of punishing them, perhaps you forgive and move on.

> Example: Remember a time when [Your Dog's Name] did something naughty, but instead of getting angry, you gently corrected them and gave them another chance. That's mercy: holding back a consequence out of love. Mercy reflects God's patience with us.

How God Shows Us Grace and Mercy (and How It Relates to Your Dog)

Similar to how your dog doesn't have to "earn" your affection, we also don't need to earn God's love or blessings. He graciously offers us His grace, even in our shortcomings. Imagine if God handed out blessings like you hand out treats to your dog, not because they're perfect, but because you delight in giving to them. When we mess up, God doesn't punish us as we deserve. Instead, He shows mercy, forgiving us and giving us another chance to grow. Your dog may not always behave perfectly, but instead of holding it against them, you offer love and forgiveness. That's how God treats us, too!

> **FUN FACT**
>
> Dachshunds were originally bred to fight badgers.
>
> Dogs that have been spayed or neutered live longer than intact dogs.

"Grace and Mercy in Action"

Step 1: Reflect on your own experiences with [Your Dog's Name]. Write down two examples:

A time you showed grace (giving them something good they didn't deserve).

A time you showed mercy (withholding a consequence they did deserve).

Step 2: Reflect on how God has shown grace and mercy to you. Write down:

A moment when you received God's grace, a blessing you didn't deserve.

A moment when you experienced God's mercy when He forgave you or withheld judgment.

Step 3: Make it practical. How can you use what you've learned to show more grace and mercy in your daily interactions with both people and [Your Dog's Name]?

The Treat of Grace

Hebrews 4:16 – "Let us then approach God's throne of grace with confidence, so that we may receive mercy and find grace to help us in our time of need."

Story: The Treat of Grace

It was one of those days when everything felt off. Exhausted and frustrated, Sarah returned home from work. Deadlines were piling up at her job, and she felt inadequate in every aspect of her life. As she stepped through the door, she barely acknowledged Max, her Labrador, who bounded towards her with enthusiasm.

"Not now, Max," Sarah sighed, dropping her bag on the floor. Nevertheless, Max wasn't dissuaded. He circled around her, tail wagging, gazing up at her with hopeful eyes.

Max had one thing on his mind: treats. Despite Sarah's tone and her distracted demeanor, he knew a simple word could change everything. With a loud bark, he sat before her, waiting eagerly.

Sarah couldn't help but chuckle. "You're something else, Max. Alright, treat."

The moment he heard that, Max dashed toward the kitchen. His joy was contagious as he twirled in excitement, eagerly anticipating the treat he knew was coming. Watching him, Sarah felt her frustration dissolve. She realized how much Max's enthusiasm reflected her own need for grace. Even on her toughest days, when she felt undeserving, exhausted, or annoyed, God's grace was always present, just waiting for her to reach out. Just as she loved giving Max a treat, God enjoyed showering her with His love and mercy.

The Lesson: Grace is Always Available

Much like Max excitedly dashed toward his treat, confident that it would be offered no matter his actions, we too can confidently approach God's throne of grace. His grace is not something we earn; it is a gift freely bestowed. Regardless of our shortcomings or feelings of unworthiness, God's grace remains accessible. We only need to approach Him with faith.

Dogs do not hesitate when they hear the word "treat." They do not question whether they deserve it, or worry about their previous behavior. They simply run with excitement, trusting in the giver. In the same way, God wants us to run to Him -- not hesitantly but confidently, knowing that He delights in pouring out His grace upon us.

RECOGNIZING GOD'S GRACE

Sometimes, we overlook God's grace because we're searching for big, miraculous signs. In reality, His grace often shows up in simple, everyday moments.

Take the following two pages to reflect on some of the following prompts:

1. List Moments of Grace:

> Take a moment to reflect on times in your life when you have felt undeserved kindness or blessings. Write these moments down, even the small ones.
>
> Examples might include:
>
> A kind word from a friend when you needed it most.
>
> A sudden sense of peace during a stressful situation.
>
> The way your dog greets you at the door, reminding you of unconditional love.

2. Daily Grace Journal:

> For the next week, keep a "Grace Journal." Each evening, write down three ways you noticed God's grace that day. These could include:

A parking spot opened up when you were in a rush.

A moment of laughter that lightened your heart.

The joy of your dog's presence brings you comfort and companionship.

3. Treat Grace as a Gift:

Just as you enjoy giving your dog treats, think about how God enjoys blessing you. Take a moment to thank Him for even the smallest blessings you receive each day.

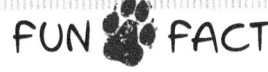

FUN FACT

More than half of all U.S. presidents have owned dogs.

Stray dogs in Russia navigate the subway system, stopping at specific locations for food.

JOURNAL NOTES

JOURNAL NOTES

Examples of God's Grace in Everyday Life

A Serene Dawn:

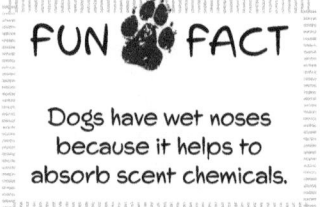

Dogs have wet noses because it helps to absorb scent chemicals.

> You rise early to witness the first light of day. It is tranquil and soothing, reminding you of God's faithfulness in granting new mercies each morning.

A Soothing Friend:

> After a long, tough day, your dog snuggles beside you. Their quiet companionship conveys so much, reassuring you that you are not alone.

Strength in Vulnerability:

> You may feel ill-equipped for a challenge, but still, you manage to persevere. God's grace frequently manifests as resilience when we require it the most.

Forgiveness:

> Maybe you yelled at your dog out of frustration, and they immediately forgave you, wagging their tail as if to say, "It's okay." This reflects the unending grace God shows us.

Surprising Happiness:

> A delightful moment shared with your dog, whether it's a silly bark, a funny trick, or their sheer excitement upon seeing you, reminds us that joy is a divine gift, even during challenging days.

LET'S JOURNAL

Take the next 2-3 pages to answer the following questions.

- When was the last time you felt overwhelmed by God's grace? Describe that moment.
- How does [Your Dog's Name]'s eagerness for treats remind you of how you should approach God's grace?
- Write about a recent moment where you may have overlooked God's grace. How can you become more aware of it in the future?

— A GIFT FROM GOD —

- What small blessings in your life, like the joy your dog brings, remind you of God's goodness?

- How can you make an intentional effort to run to God's grace with the same confidence and excitement that your dog shows when running for a treat?

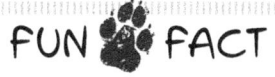

FUN FACT

Does your dog have separation anxiety? Leave some of your worn clothing with him. The scent can help ease his anxiety.

JOURNAL NOTES

JOURNAL NOTES

JOURNAL NOTES

CLOSING REFLECTION

Grace is a gift that is always available, no matter what. Just like your dog runs eagerly to you for treats, you can confidently approach God, knowing His grace is waiting for you. Take a moment to thank Him for the ways He's shown you grace today through your dog, through quiet moments, and through the blessings you may not have noticed before.

A LETTER FROM GOD TO [YOUR DOG'S NAME]

Take the following two pages to write a letter as if it's from God to [Your Dog's Name]. In this letter, God is instructing your dog to love, protect, and bring joy to their owner.

> Example: "Dear [Your Dog's Name],
>
> Thank you for being the joy-filled soul that lights up [Owner's Name]'s life. I created you with a wagging tail to bring happiness and a loving heart to remind them of My love every day. Keep being the amazing companion I made you to be!"

Reflection: This activity helps readers reflect on their dog's role as a blessing while connecting back to God's care and intentionality.

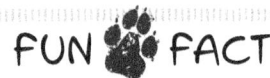

FUN FACT

Your dog can sense your feelings. Their sense of smell is about 100,000 times better than yours, allowing them to detect emotions, like fear, through perspiration change.

Dogs can detect cancer and other diseases in humans by sniffing out the metabolic waste of cancerous cells, even in a person's breath.

JOURNAL NOTES

JOURNAL NOTES

— FUR-EVER FRIENDS —

EVERY JOURNEY STARTS WITH A SINGLE STEP

The Journey to Being Blessed with [Your Dog's Name]:

In the following page, take some time to map out your dog's story. This is your chance to be creative and celebrate the special bond you share with your furry companion! Use the questions below to guide you and express your love for [Your Dog's Name]:

- Where were you the first time you saw [Your Dog's Name]?
- How did you feel when you realized they were going to be yours?
- What do you think God showed you by bringing [Your Dog's Name] into your life?

Add your personal touch:

- Draw a picture of the day [Your Dog's Name] came home. Paste a favorite photo of you and [Your Dog's Name].

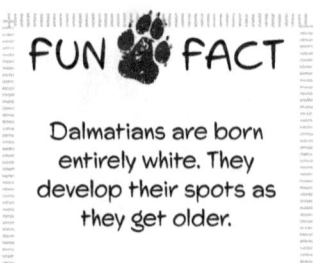

FUN FACT

Dalmatians are born entirely white. They develop their spots as they get older.

JOURNAL NOTES

LET'S JOURNAL

Take the following 2-3 pages to answer the questions below.

1. Reflect on how [Your Dog's Name] became a part of your life.

    Can you see God's hand in bringing them to you? How did this moment feel like a blessing?

2. List three things you love most about [Your Dog's Name].

    What makes them unique and special in your eyes?

3. Share a time when [Your Dog's Name] brought you unexpected joy or comfort.

    Was it a quiet cuddle, a playful antic, or a moment that reminded you everything would be okay?

4. Consider how [Your Dog's Name] reflects God's love and provision.

    What about their presence reminds you of God's faithfulness and care?

5. Celebrate what makes [Your Dog's Name] so perfect for you.

    Why do you feel they are the ideal companion for your life?

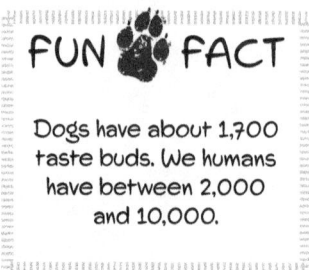

FUN FACT

Dogs have about 1,700 taste buds. We humans have between 2,000 and 10,000.

JOURNAL NOTES

JOURNAL NOTES

JOURNAL NOTES

— FUR-EVER FRIENDS —

A POEM FOR [YOUR DOG'S NAME]

Psalm 36:6 – "You, Lord, preserve both people and animals."

Oh, [Your Dog's Name], a gift beyond compare,

A blessing from God, so tender and rare.

Your wagging tail and playful cheer,

Fill my days with joy, year after year.

You teach me to love without an end,

Not just a pet, but my dearest friend.

Through you, God's grace shines pure and true,

A reflection of His love in all that you do.

Can you create a poem about [Your Dog's Name]?

Philippians 4:13 – I can do all things through Christ who strengthens me.

Use the following two pages to craft a poem about [Your Dog's Name]. Reflect on the memories in this book, or think of new experiences you've had with your furry friend. Just as our Creator embodies creativity, He also instills that same gift in you and your dog.

Take a moment to explore that creative spirit. You might surprise yourself with what comes forth about your canine companion. Remember, it's not about crafting perfect rhymes; this exercise is an avenue for heartfelt expression and gratitude toward your dog(s).

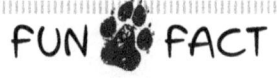

FUN FACT

When dogs kick backward after they go to the bathroom, it's not to cover up the urine but to mark their territory, using the scent glands in their feet.

A study shows that dogs are among a small group of animals who show voluntary, unselfish kindness towards others without any reward.

JOURNAL NOTES

JOURNAL NOTES

HOW WELL DO YOU KNOW YOUR DOG'S FAVORITE FOODS?

Here is a list of food items. Pick five of your dog's favorite foods.

Corn	Zucchini	Watermelon	Lettuce
Lamb	Eggs	Blueberries	Pumpkin
Blackberries	Brussels sprouts	Potatoes	Turkey
Peas	Bananas	Green Beans	Cabbage
Liver	Kale	Cucumber	Beef
Pear	Pork	Carrots	Apples
Sweet Potatoes	Spinach	Celery	
Fish	Sardines	Broccoli	

PAW PRINT GRATITUDE KEEPSAKE

A dog's paw print acts as a signature of their presence in your life, evoking the unique joy and companionship they offer. This activity enables you to create a lovely, tangible keepsake of your dog's paw, accompanied by heartfelt words of appreciation that convey their importance to you. It transcends a mere craft; it become a spiritual practice that recognizes God's blessings and shares that gratitude with others.

How to Create Your Paw Print Keepsake

What You'll Need:

- Safe, non-toxic pet paint or a paw print kit (available at pet stores or online).

- Thick paper, canvas, or cardstock for the keepsake.

- Washable wet wipes or a damp cloth to clean your dog's paw.

- Markers, pens, or decorative items (e.g., stickers, glitter, or washi tape).

- A quiet, comfortable space for you and your dog.

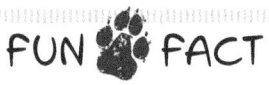

FUN FACT

Cheetahs can run faster than Greyhounds, reaching 70 mph for thirty seconds. However, Greyhounds maintain 35 mph over seven miles and eventually overtake cheetahs.

Prepare Your Space:

> Lay down an old towel or plastic sheet to protect your workspace. Ensure your dog is relaxed, perhaps after a walk or playtime, so they are calm and cooperative.

Apply the Paint:

> Gently apply a thin layer of safe, non-toxic paint to your dog's paw. Use a soft brush or sponge to ensure even coverage.

Make the Print:

> Press your dog's paw gently onto the paper or canvas. Hold it steady for a moment, then lift their paw straight up to avoid smudging.

Clean Up:

> Immediately clean your dog's paw with wet wipes or a damp cloth to remove any remaining paint. Praise them for being such a good helper!

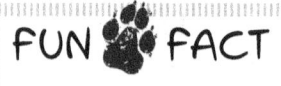

FUN FACT

Dogs often choose spots to poop aligned with the Earth's magnetic field.

Add Gratitude Words:

> Around the paw print, write words or phrases that express your gratitude for your dog and the blessings they bring. Examples: Joy-bringer, God's gift, My comforter, Unconditional love, Faithful friend

Decorate:

Use markers,stickers, or other decorations to personalize your keepsake. You could include your dog's name, their birth or adoption date, or a favorite Bible verse (e.g., Psalm 36:6: "You, Lord, preserve both people and animals").

Frame It (Optional):

> Once it's dry, frame the keepsake to display in your home or give as a gift.

How to Use the Keepsake

1. Display It at Home:

> Hang the paw print in a special spot where you'll see it often—perhaps near your dog's favorite place to nap or in your prayer corner. Let it serve as a daily reminder of God's blessings.

2. Use It as a Gift:

> For Family or Friends: Create one for someone who loves your dog (e.g., a family member or friend who pet sits). It's a heartfelt, personal gift that shares the joy your dog brings.
>
> For a Fellow Dog Lover: Encourage someone else to see God's blessings through their own dog by gifting them a paw print from your dog along with a note of gratitude for their companionship.

3. Share God's Love:

> Include a small card with a scripture verse, such as Isaiah 43:20 or Proverbs 12:10, explaining how your dog reflects God's care and love. This can be a meaningful way to share your faith with others.

4. Create a Keepsake Collection:

> If you have multiple dogs or pets, make a keepsake for each one. Over time, you'll have a collection that celebrates all the animals God has placed in your life.

How to Use It Spiritually

Gratitude Journal Add-On:

> Place the keepsake in your journal or scrapbook. Use it as a starting point to write prayers of thanksgiving for your dog and the blessings they bring to your life.

Reflection Tool:

> Spend time reflecting on the words of gratitude you have written around the paw print. Think about how your dog's loyalty, joy, and comfort reflect God's character.

Prayer Aid:

> When you see the keepsake, say a prayer of thanks for your dog and ask God to help you show the same love and care to all of His creation.

LET'S HAVE SOME FUN!

Family Collaboration:

> If you have kids or family members, involve them in the process. Each person can write their own words of gratitude around the paw print to create a collaborative family keepsake.

Seasonal Paw Prints:

> Make themed keepsakes for holidays or seasons. For example, a Christmas paw print with the phrase "God's Christmas blessing" or a summer-themed keepsake with "God's sunshine in my life."

Align Your Handprint with Your Dog's:

> Place your handprint alongside your dog's paw print to represent your connection and collaboration. Beneath the prints, jot down a meaningful prayer or scripture that reflects your shared journey.

CLOSING REFLECTION

This paw print keepsake is not just a craft; it reflects God's creativity, love, and intentionality in placing [Your Dog's Name] in your life. Each time you see it, let it remind you of the unique joy your dog brings and the God who loves you enough to bless you with their companionship.

HE'S ALWAYS WORKING ON OUR BEHALF!

Below are two stories where dogs serve as instruments of God to save lives. These accounts merely scratch the surface of how dogs have selflessly supported their human companions. This is not mere coincidence: each of these occurrences has significance, and God can and will act through our pets to achieve that significance. As you delve into these stories, I invite you to contemplate your own experiences with your dog and think about how they may have saved you, perhaps even from yourself

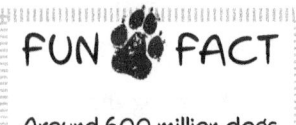

FUN FACT

Around 600 million dogs globally exist, with an estimated 400 million being strays.

Dog Saves a Three-Year-Old Girl

In 2017, a dog rescued from an abusive owner found a loving home and became a hero. Peanut, a once-abandoned dog, alerted her family with intense barking about danger outside their house. While searching for her in freezing conditions, her family was shocked to discover a hypothermic 3-year-old girl on the brink of death, who had reportedly fled from an abusive home by herself. Peanut's loud commotion that day ultimately saved the little girl's life.

Dog Saved His Owner from Freezing to Death

Grga Brkić was ascending the highest peak in Croatia's Velebit mountain range, towering around 5,800 feet above the Adriatic coast, when he fell approximately 500 feet down a snowy slope. The fall inflicted a severe fracture on Brkić's leg.

Nearby hikers noticed Brkić and his companion, an Alaskan malamute, but could not safely approach. As Brkić shivered on the ground, his dog lay on top of him to provide warmth until help arrived. After enduring 13 hours in the freezing temperatures, the responders were astonished to see that the dog had curled around Brkić to keep him warm.

CLOSING THOUGHT

Your dog's talent for providing comfort is a divine gift, showcasing God's love and care. Like God, who is near to the brokenhearted, He has given [Your Dog's Name] to you as a physical manifestation of His presence. Cherish these restorative moments, allowing them to bring you nearer to the One who loves you beyond measure.

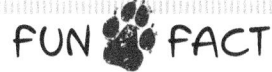

FUN FACT

Michael Vick's former dogs, Sox and Hector, are certified therapy dogs that cheer people in hospitals, nursing homes, and schools.

Spiked collars were originally fashioned in ancient Greece to protect dogs' throats from wolf attacks.

The Bloodhound's sense of smell is so accurate that its tracking results can be used as court evidence law.

— FUR-EVER FRIENDS —

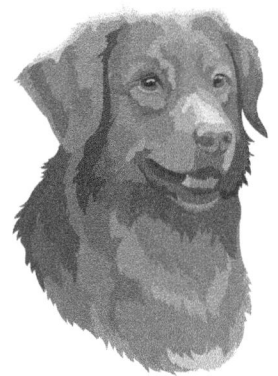

CHAPTER 11:
Love Without Words

1 John 4:19 – "We love because He first loved us."

FOOD FOR THOUGHT?

Have you ever observed how your dog shows affection without saying anything? A wagging tail, a gentle nuzzle, or a soft lick on your hand conveys deep emotions. Dogs do not require words to demonstrate their love. Their actions are genuine, straightforward, and constant. This mirrors the beauty of God's love for us, which is silent yet unwavering, unspoken yet unconditional, and always there.

True love is not dependent on words; it can be seen, felt, and experienced in those quiet moments, and in how your dog curls up next to you, watching your every move and eagerly standing by the door waiting for you. These simple, silent gestures of loyalty reflect God's immense love for His children, shown through deeds rather than words.

EXPLORING LOVE WITHOUT WORDS

The Greeks had four words to describe the word "love":

1. Agape – Unconditional, selfless love.

2. Philia – Brotherly love or deep friendship.

3. Storge – Familial love, the bond of kinship.

4. Eros – Romantic love.

Our dogs embody a beautiful combination of Agape and Storge love. They show us unconditional affection and completely accept our imperfections. To them, we are everything, and they give their loyalty and love freely, asking for nothing in return.

Dogs love without any judgment. Their actions demonstrate how to love others selflessly, reflecting how God loves us. Just as we appreciate our dogs in their quiet moments, God values us in ours. He perceives our hearts even when we cannot express them, meeting us in life's stillness with His endless love and compassion.

Examples of Loving Without Words

Silent Comforter:

> Picture a day when you felt down, and your dog quietly rested their head on your lap. No words were needed; their presence spoke volumes, saying, "I'm here for you." This simple act mirrors the way God comforts us in silence, reminding us that we are never alone.

Joyful Greeting:

> After a long day, your dog rushes to the door, tail wagging with pure excitement. They don't need to say, "I missed you," because their actions speak for themselves. It is a beautiful reflection of how God welcomes us back with open arms, no matter how far we have strayed.

Unwavering Loyalty:

> Your dog follows you from room to room, content to be near you. This quiet loyalty reflects God's promise to always be by our side, a constant presence that never leaves or forsakes us.

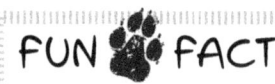

FUN FACT

Guinness World Records recognizes Zeus, a Great Dane, as the tallest male dog at 3 feet, 5.18 inches.

According to Guinness World Records, Pearl the Chihuahua is the shortest dog ever recorded, measuring 3.59 inches tall.

WHAT DOES LOVE LOOK LIKE?

Take the following two pages and reflect on how love expresses itself in action between you and your dog.

- If your dog could not wag their tail, lick your hand, or cuddle with you, how else might they show their love?

- How would you show your love to [Your Dog's Name] if you couldn't use words?

This activity invites you to focus on the heart behind your and your dog's actions, celebrating the unspoken bond that connects you both.

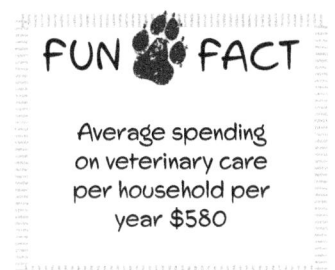

FUN FACT

Average spending on veterinary care per household per year $580

JOURNAL NOTES

JOURNAL NOTES

— FUR-EVER FRIENDS —

LET'S JOURNAL

Take the following 2-3 pages to answer the following questions below.

1. Share a moment when [Your Dog's Name] demonstrated love without words.

    How did their actions make you feel?

2. Reflect on the quiet moments you shared with [Your Dog's Name].

    What do those moments teach you about God's love?

3. Think about how [Your Dog's Name] comforts you.

    How do they show care when you're feeling upset or tired?

4. Consider showing [Your Dog's Name] love without words.

    What actions could express your love in ways they would understand?

5. Write about a time when you felt God's presence in silence.

    How does that experience compare to the way your dog shows love?

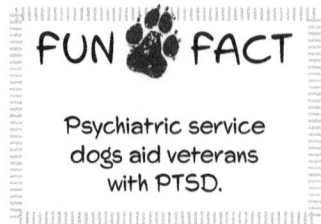

FUN FACT

Psychiatric service dogs aid veterans with PTSD.

JOURNAL NOTES

JOURNAL NOTES

JOURNAL NOTES

A DAY OF SILENT LOVE

Take the following 2-3 pages to answer the questions below.

Spend a day observing how [Your Dog's Name] shows their love for you in ways not mentioned in this book. Taking the time to notice could uncover many examples. Pay attention to every moment, whether it is a slight wag of their tail, a gentle resting of their head on your knee, or simply their comforting presence in the same room. These are just a few suggestions, and I invite you to think of other moments to record, as we all have so much to share about the quiet affection our dogs give us. Sometimes, silence is crucial for us to appreciate the blessings we have received or the obstacles we have overcome. Often, we hear God's voice most clearly when we silence distractions and take a moment to reflect.

Document these instances as they happen, then take a moment to ponder: How do these subtle, silent expressions of love mirror how God quietly demonstrates His love for you?

If possible, consider taking your dog somewhere outside your home, like a park, beach, or a new walking trail during this time.

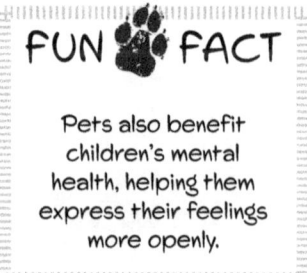

JOURNAL NOTES

JOURNAL NOTES

JOURNAL NOTES

HE'S ALWAYS WORKING ON OUR BEHALF

Below are two stories of moments when dogs served as instruments of God to save lives. "The following stories share moments when dogs became God's hands and feet, stepping in to save lives. They offer just a glimpse of the many ways our canine companions have shown extraordinary devotion and courage. I don't believe these moments happen by chance; each one carries meaning, a reminder that God can work through our pets in remarkable ways. As you read, consider your journey with your dog and reflect on the times they may have rescued you, perhaps even from struggles within yourself.

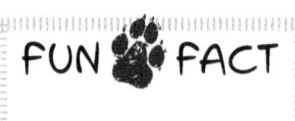

FUN FACT

The Australian Shepherd is not actually from Australia. In fact, they are an American breed.

A Dog Saves a Choking Woman

Debbie Parkhurst was startled when she began choking on an apple. Just as she was trying to figure out how to save herself, her dog Toby jumped onto her chest. The American Society for the Prevention of Cruelty to Animals (ASPCA) recognized the Golden Retriever with an award for his heroic rescue efforts.

Dog Saved Its Owner from a Venomous Snake

While hiking, Paula Godwin nearly stepped on a venomous rattlesnake. Fortunately, her one-year-old dog intervened to save her. As the snake lunged, Todd bravely positioned himself in front of her and was bitten on the nose in the process. He was rushed to a local veterinary hospital for treatment, with Godwin by his side. Todd's act of bravery captured significant attention online, leading various organizations to assist with his medical expenses.

CLOSING THOUGHT

Dogs teach us that love transcends words; it is about being there. Their silent affection mirrors God's agape love: steadfast, unspoken, and unconditional. While you reflect on [Your Dog's Name] and the distinct ways they express their devotion, consider the subtle ways God shows His love and care for you daily.

"Though the mountains be shaken and the hills be removed, yet my unfailing love for you will not be shaken." – Isaiah 54:10

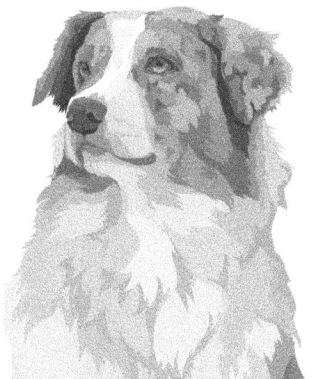

CHAPTER III:
Companionship in Every Season

Joshua 1:9 – "Be strong and courageous. Do not be afraid; do not be discouraged, for the Lord your God will be with you wherever you go."

WHAT IS COMPANIONSHIP?

Companionship is one of life's most profound gifts, a blessing from God that assures us of our shared existence. At its essence, companionship involves being there for each other in all circumstances, whether in times of joy, hardship or everything in-between. God recognizes our desire for connection and often meets that need through our relationships with others, including the special bond you have with your dog.

Your dog is a daily reminder of God's promise to accompany you consistently. Every time your dog curls up beside you or matches your steps, it's a small echo of a greater truth: God is near. Their quiet loyalty mirrors His promise never to leave you, walking with you through every joy, every challenge, and every in-between moment. Just as

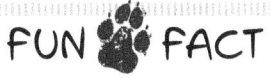

FUN 🐾 FACT

Pets Foster Connection and Community

Pets Reduce Feelings of Loneliness

your dog loyally walks beside you, God desires to accompany you through every phase of your life.

UNDERSTANDING "SEASONS" IN LIFE

Life unfolds in seasons, each bringing its challenges and joys. Here are some ways these seasons connect to companionship, especially the bond you share with your dog:

1. Spring: New Beginnings

> Spring is a season of growth, excitement, and fresh starts. It is like when you first brought [Your Dog's Name] home. Those early days were filled with joy and discovery but also came with challenges, like training or getting to know your dog's personality.
>
> For example, think of the first time [Your Dog's Name] wagged their tail at you or mastered a command. This season reminds us that growth takes patience and that God walks with us every step of the way.

2. Summer: Joy and Abundance

> Summer represents the high points of laughter, play, and abundance. It is those moments when your dog runs freely in the yard or leaps excitedly when you grab their leash for a walk.
>
> For example, picture a sunny day when you and [Your Dog's Name] played fetch or went on an adventure together. These moments reflect God's desire for us to experience joy and fullness in His presence.

4. Autumn: Change and Reflection

> Autumn is a season of change and gratitude. It is when your dog begins to mature, and your bond with them deepens. This is a time to reflect on the little things that bring meaning to life.
>
> For example, recall a quiet moment shared with [Your Dog's Name], sitting together as the leaves fell, simply enjoying their presence. Like your dog's companionship, God's love remains a constant through seasons of change.

5. Winter: Challenges and Stillness

> Winter symbolizes hardship and stillness. Perhaps it was when [Your Dog's Name] was sick or when you faced a difficult decision about their care. This season teaches us the value of companionship during life's storms.
>
> For example, consider when [Your Dog's Name] sat quietly beside you, offering comfort on a tough day. Just as your dog provides peace and strength, God's presence wraps us in His unwavering love during life's challenges.

Conversations about pets over fences sometimes led to gatherings, especially when neighborhood children wanted to meet new pets.

Types of Companionship

Companionship comes in many forms, and your dog might fulfill multiple roles in your life:

Acquaintance:

> The early days of your relationship with [Your Dog's Name], when you were beginning to learn each other's quirks, habits, and personalities.

Casual Friend:

> The simple joy of sharing playful moments like tossing a ball, teaching a trick, or enjoying a carefree walk together.

Close Friend:

> The comfort of familiarity, knowing [Your Dog's Name] 's routines, and feeling uplifted by their daily presence.

Confidant:

> The trust grows when your dog senses your emotions and responds with quiet, unwavering support.

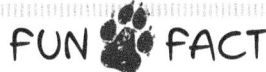

FUN FACT

Dog parents reported high social interaction, with 27% of pet owners meeting neighbors through their animals.

A study found that pets in the classroom enhance social skills and reading competence while reducing hyperactivity. Parents noted their children became more empathetic and caring at home.

Soulmate-like Connection:

> That indescribable bond where [Your Dog's Name] feels like a piece of your soul, a reflection of God's deep desire to connect with you similarly.

God yearns for a soulmate-like bond with you. Your dog's companionship provides a glimpse into the deep, unconditional love and connection He wishes to share with you.

COMFORT AND JOY

Comfort:

> The quiet peace that comes from simply having your dog by your side. It's the weight of their head on your lap when you're feeling down or their steady gaze that seems to say, "I'm here for you."

Joy:

> The pure burst of happiness from their wagging tail, playful bark, or silly antics, which makes you smile even on the most challenging days.

Reflection:

Can you think of a moment when [Your Dog's Name] brought you both comfort and joy? Take some time to reflect and write it down below!

God uses our dogs to provide comfort and joy, reminding us of His love and care in unique and beautiful ways.

FUN 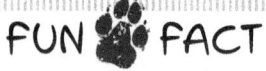 FACT

Dogs encourage Mindfulness and focus

Dog health benefits go beyond walks; interactions release oxytocin, endorphins, and prolactin in humans, reducing cortisol. Your pet experiences positive changes too.

COMPANIONSHIP REFLECTION

Take the following 2-3 pages to answer the questions below.

If [Your Dog's Name] could write you a letter, what would they say about how you show them companionship and love?

Now, imagine God writing you a letter. What would He say about how He has shown you companionship and care?

This activity invites you to reflect on the flow of love and presence from you to your dog and from God to you. Take your time, and be completely honest in your responses.

/ JOURNAL NOTES

JOURNAL NOTES

JOURNAL NOTES

— COMPANIONSHIP IN EVERY SEASON —

LET'S JOURNAL

Take the following 2-3 pages to answer the questions below.

1. Describe a season when [Your Dog's Name] brought you comfort.

    How did they show their companionship during that time?

2. Reflect on a joyful moment with [Your Dog's Name].

    How did this experience remind you of God's goodness?

3. Think about a challenging season in your life.

    How was [Your Dog's Name] there for you then?

4. What qualities in [Your Dog's Name] remind you of God's companionship?

    How do these traits reflect His love and care for you?

5. Consider the season of life you're in now.

    How does [Your Dog's Name] bring you comfort or joy in this moment?

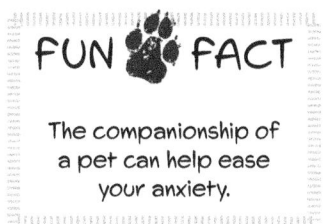

The companionship of a pet can help ease your anxiety.

JOURNAL NOTES

— COMPANIONSHIP IN EVERY SEASON —

JOURNAL NOTES

JOURNAL NOTES

HE IS ALWAYS WORKING ON OUR BEHALF!

Below are stories of times when dogs served as instruments of God to save lives. Some moments with dogs stop us in our tracks, not because they're cute or funny, but because they reveal something sacred. In the pages ahead, you'll read about times when a dog's actions meant the difference between life and death. I believe these moments aren't random. They are glimpses of God at work through our four-legged friends. As you take in these stories, think back to your own life. Has your dog ever been more than a companion, perhaps even a quiet hero who helped save you in ways you didn't expect?

Dog Saves a Little Boy from a Cougar

Eleven-year-old Austin Forman was playing in his yard when a cougar suddenly emerged and attacked him. As the cougar charged, his dog leaped in front of him, preventing the attack. The brave 18-month-old Golden Retriever fought valiantly against the larger animal, giving Austin a chance to escape to safety. The family quickly called 911, and a police officer shot and killed the cougar.

The brave dog named Angel suffered serious injuries but made a full recovery. Today, she spends her days with her thankful family, including the young boy who understands he has a furry guardian angel watching over him.

A Dog Sacrificed His Life for the Police

German Shepherd Diesel was a Belgian Shepherd serving with the French police. While on a search, Diesel discovered the apartment of a suspect involved in the Paris terrorist attack. He suffered multiple gunshot wounds from the assailant and ultimately succumbed to his injuries. Diesel's bravery saved the lives of his police colleagues. In recognition of his sacrifice, he was awarded the Dickin Medal and featured in Time magazine's 2016 list of the world's most influential animals. His memory will live on in the hearts and minds of people everywhere in the world.

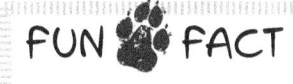

Three dogs survived the historical sinking of the Titanic in 1912. Two Pomeranians and 1 Pekingese - all from First Class cabins.

Seven Daily Affirmations Based on Scripture

1. "You are my gift from God. I treasure you as He treasures me." (**James 1:17**)

2. "Your love reminds me of God's constant care." (**Joshua 1:9**)

3. "You are fearfully and wonderfully made by God." (**Psalm 139:14**)

4. "Your companionship reflects God's love for me." (**1 John 4:19**)

5. "I am grateful for you every day as a sign of God's provision." (**Psalm 36:6**)

6. "Through you, I see God's faithfulness in every season." (**Ecclesiastes 3:1**)

7. "You are my blessing, a reminder of God's unchanging love." (**Lamentations 3:22-23**)

FUN 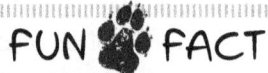 FACT

Pets can significantly boost self-confidence. They are excellent listeners and provide unconditional love free from judgment. This kind of support is especially valuable when one feels lonely or misjudged.

All Dogs Are Directly Descended from Wolves

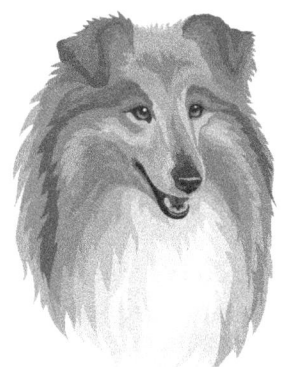

CHAPTER IV:

Lessons from [Your Dog's Name]

Proverbs 12:10 – "The righteous care for the needs of their animals."

DOGS AS TEACHERS OF GODLY VIRTUES

Have you ever taken a moment to reflect on the lessons your dog has imparted? God communicates through the simple, quiet interactions with [Your Dog's Name]. Each wag of their tail, a gentle nudge, or playful bark carries a significant message if we pause to listen.

This chapter encourages you to uncover your dog's lessons about love, patience, responsibility, resilience, and more.

In His boundless wisdom, God employs the animals in our lives to nurture virtues we might not otherwise learn. As the righteous care for their pets, animals also care for us. Their steadfast love and companionship remind us of God's continual provision and His desire to shape our hearts and characters.

LESSONS FROM YOUR DOG, CONNECTED TO GOD

Responsibility

Caring for [Your Dog's Name] teaches us to be consistent, dependable, and intentional. Whether we feed them at the same time each day, take them on walks, or ensure their health, this responsibility mirrors God's care for us.

> Example: Think of the mornings when [Your Dog's Name] patiently (or excitedly) waits for their breakfast, trusting that you will provide. Just as they rely on you, we can rely on God to meet our daily needs.
>
> Scriptural Connection:
>
> *Philippians 4:19 – "And my God will meet all your needs according to the riches of his glory in Christ Jesus."*

Unconditional Love

Dogs do not judge you based on your mistakes or stormy days; they love you just as you are. As we've discussed, their unwavering love reflects God's agape love: unconditional and constant.

> Example: Recall a time when you felt down, and [Your Dog's Name] quietly stayed by your side. Their comforting presence mirrors the steadfast love God shows us.
>
> Scriptural Connection:
>
> *Romans 8:38-39 – "Nothing can separate us from the love of God."*

Empathy

Dogs sense our emotions and respond with care. Their ability to connect with us can teach us to develop empathy for others.

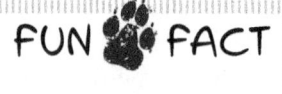

FUN FACT

Maltese dogs do not shed, making them perfect pups for people with allergies.

> Example: When you are upset, [Your Dog's Name] might nuzzle you or stay close. This reflects God's call for us to bear one another's burdens.

Scriptural Connection:

Galatians 6:2 – "Carry each other's burdens, and in this way, you will fulfill the law of Christ."

Patience

Training and caring for a dog both require patience and understanding. It takes time for them to learn and grow, just as it takes time for us to develop in our faith.

> FUN  FACT
>
> Puppies and kittens can be adopted as early as 8 weeks of age. Until then, they should stay with their moms and littermates.
>
> A Dog's Nose Is Its Fingerprint

> Example: Think about the time and effort it took to teach [Your Dog's Name] a command like "sit" or "stay." This process mirrors God's patient guidance as we grow spiritually.

Scriptural Connection:

Psalm 86:15 – "But you, Lord, are a compassionate and gracious God, slow to anger, abounding in love and faithfulness."

Resilience

Dogs are incredibly resilient, returning from challenges like injuries, fears, or new environments. They remind us that setbacks do not define us.

> Example: Perhaps [Your Dog's Name] faced a health scare or overcame a fear with your support. Their resilience reflects God's promise to strengthen and uphold us.

Scriptural Connection:

Isaiah 41:10 – "So do not fear, for I am with you; do not be dismayed, for I am your God. I will strengthen you and help you."

Trust Wisely

Your dog instinctively trusts you to care for them but remains cautious in unfamiliar situations. This teaches us the importance of discerning whom we trust.

Example: [Your Dog's Name] might hesitate before approaching a stranger but runs to you without hesitation. This reminds us to place our ultimate trust in God, who is always faithful.

Scriptural Connection:

Proverbs 3:5 – "Trust in the Lord with all your heart and lean not on your own understanding."

Love Without Conditions

Dogs do not care about your appearance, status, or mistakes; their love is not dependent on these things.

> Example: After a hard day, when you feel at your lowest, [Your Dog's Name] still wags their tail and shows you affection.

Scriptural Connection:

> **FUN FACT**
> Over 150 dog breeds are divided into 8 classes: sporting, hound, working, terrier, toy, non-sporting, herding, and miscellaneous.

1 John 4:8 – "Whoever does not love does not know God, because God is love."

Balance Work and Play

Dogs are masters of living with balance; they rest peacefully yet are always ready for action when needed. Similarly, : God calls us to work diligently, rest, and enjoy His creation.

Example: [Your Dog's Name] might relax by your side but springs to life when it is time for a walk or playtime.

Scriptural Connection:

Ecclesiastes 3:1 – "There is a time for everything and a season for every activity under the heavens."

Be Present for Those You Love

Your dog is always tuned in to you, watching, waiting, and responding to your emotions.

Example: [Your Dog's Name] knows when you feel happy or sad and acts accordingly. This reminds us to be attentive and present for the people we care about.

Scriptural Connection:

Romans 12:10 – "Be devoted to one another in love. Honor one another above yourselves."

Trust That It Will Be Okay

Dogs have a way of living fully in the moment, never burdened by what tomorrow might bring. They believe their needs will be met.

Example: During a thunderstorm, [Your Dog's Name] trembles at the first rumble of thunder, then dashes to your side. With one look into your eyes, they seem to know they're safe. That simple act of trust mirrors the way God invites us to run to Him in our fear, believing He will hold us steady until the storm passes.

Scriptural Connection:

Isaiah 26:3-4 (NIV) – "You will keep in perfect peace those whose minds are steadfast, because they trust in you. Trust in the Lord forever, for the Lord, the Lord himself, is the Rock eternal."

Embrace Who You Were Created to Be

Your dog never tries to be anything other than themselves; they live fully as God designed them to be. Just as God created your dog to be exactly who they are, He created you to be uniquely you. Embracing who you are is part of living out His plan.

Example: [Your Dog's Name] barks excitedly, sniffs the ground with curiosity, and plays with toys uniquely. They do not question their purpose; they live it with joy.

Scriptural Connection:

Psalm 139:14 – "I praise you because I am fearfully and wonderfully made; your works are wonderful; I know that full well."

— FUR-EVER FRIENDS —

LESSONS PAW BY PAW

Take the following 2-3 pages to answer the questions below while reflecting on the lessons [Your Dog's Name] has taught you.

1. Write down five specific lessons they've shown you.

2. Next to each lesson, describe how [Your Dog's Name] taught it to you through their actions or behavior.

3. Find a scripture that connects to each lesson, highlighting its spiritual significance

Example

> Lesson: Patience.
>
> How [Your Dog's Name] taught it: Training your dog to sit takes time, effort, and understanding.
>
> Scripture:
>
> Psalm 86:15 – *"But you, Lord, are a compassionate and gracious God, slow to anger, abounding in love and faithfulness."*

This activity encourages you to see the deeper meanings behind your experiences with [Your Dog's Name] and connect them to God's teachings in scripture

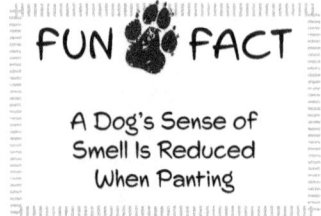

FUN FACT

A Dog's Sense of Smell Is Reduced When Panting

— LESSONS FROM [YOUR DOG'S NAME] —

JOURNAL NOTES

JOURNAL NOTES

— LESSONS FROM [YOUR DOG'S NAME] —

JOURNAL NOTES

LET'S JOURNAL

Take the following 2-3 pages to answer the questions below.

Responsibility:

Reflect on your daily routines with [Your Dog's Name].

> What have these routines taught you about being dependable?

> How have these lessons influenced other areas of your life?

Unconditional Love:

Consider a moment when [Your Dog's Name] showed you love despite your mood or actions.

> How did that moment make you feel?

> How does it remind you of God's unconditional love?

Empathy:

Consider how [Your Dog's Name] senses your emotions.

> Write about a time when they comforted you during a difficult moment.

> How did their empathy impact you?

Patience:

Think about something you had to teach [Your Dog's Name] that required a lot of patience.

> How did that experience help you grow in patience toward others?

Resilience:

Recall a challenge [Your Dog's Name] faced and overcame.

> How did their resilience inspire you to face your struggles with strength?

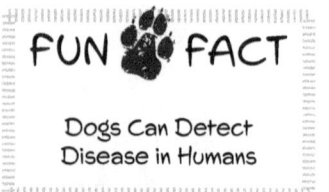

FUN FACT

Dogs Can Detect Disease in Humans

— LESSONS FROM [YOUR DOG'S NAME] —

JOURNAL NOTES

JOURNAL NOTES

— LESSONS FROM [YOUR DOG'S NAME] —

JOURNAL NOTES

FINAL REFLECTION QUESTIONS

Take the following 2-3 pages to answer the questions below.

> Which three lessons that [Your Dog's Name] has taught you stand out the most? Why are they so meaningful to you?

How have these lessons changed you as a person?

> Think about how you've grown because of your experiences with [Your Dog's Name].

What have these lessons taught you about God's care and love for you?

> Reflect on how your relationship with [Your Dog's Name] has deepened your understanding of God's character.

How can you use these lessons to bless or help others?

> Consider applying these insights to encourage and support the people around you.

If [Your Dog's Name] could understand every word you said, what would you thank them for teaching you?

> Please take a moment to express gratitude for how they've impacted your life in a way you have not described in previous questions while working on this book.

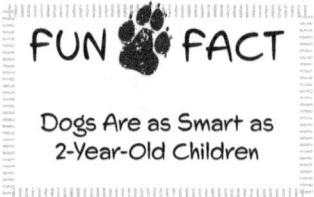

FUN FACT

Dogs Are as Smart as 2-Year-Old Children

— LESSONS FROM [YOUR DOG'S NAME] —

JOURNAL NOTES

JOURNAL NOTES

— LESSONS FROM [YOUR DOG'S NAME] —

JOURNAL NOTES

HOW MUCH HAVE YOU TAUGHT [YOUR DOG'S NAME]?

Here are some tricks that people have taught their dogs. Which trick have you taught your dog?

Spin	High-Five
Take a Bow	Stand
Pray	Teaching hush
Jump rope	Sit
Rollover	Hug
Close the door	Limp
Kiss	Teach your dog locations
Teamwork	Clean up
Speak	Tug
Lie down	Wave Peek-a-boo
Self-confidence	Open/Close the door
Turn lights on/off	Crawl
Play Dead Retrieve	Leg Weaves
Down	Get your dish
Paw (shake)	Fetch
Come	Yes and No
Eye Contact	Put toys away
Shake	Leave it
Wait	Back up
Heel	Search/find it
Kiss	Stay
Jump	Beg
Jump through hoops	Catch

HE IS ALWAYS WORKING ON OUR BEHALF!

Below are stories of times when dogs served as instruments of God to save lives. These accounts merely scratch the surface of how dogs have selflessly supported their human companions. This isn't a coincidence; I believe each occurrence has significance, and God can and will act through our pets to achieve that significance. This particularly involves our furry friends assisting in saving our lives. As you delve into these stories, I invite you to contemplate your

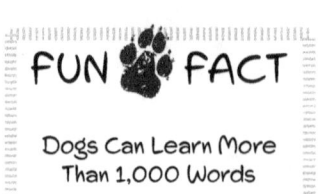

FUN FACT

Dogs Can Learn More Than 1,000 Words

own experiences with your dog and think about how they may have saved you, perhaps even from yourself.

A Blind Dog Saved a Drowning Girl

Lab Retrievers are famous for their enthusiasm for running, playing, and enjoying water, making beach outings especially fun.

Norman, a blind Labrador retriever rescued from a difficult situation, exemplified this spirit. He bravely leaped into the water to save a little girl who was nearly drowning. By attentively listening to her cries, Norman could locate her and guide her to the safe coast.

A Dog Called 911 to Save His Owner's Life

A Labrador retriever and pit bull mix named Major saved his owner, a PTSD-suffering U.S. Marine, during an impending seizure. As the owner began to seize, Major used his paw to tap on the mobile phone in his owner's pocket, attempting to call 911. Initially, dispatchers mistook the call for a prank and kept the line open. Undeterred, Major persisted in the call. Eventually, they recognized McGlade's voice and dispatched medics. Upon arrival, Major greeted them outside the building, guiding them to his owner's location.

CLOSING THOUGHT

Dogs are more than companions; they are God's gentle teachers, sent to reflect His love and virtues in ways we can see, feel, and experience daily. Each lesson from [Your Dog's Name] reminds us of God's character and allows us to grow deeper in faith and understanding.

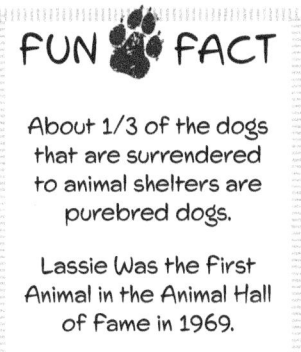

FUN FACT

About 1/3 of the dogs that are surrendered to animal shelters are purebred dogs.

Lassie Was the first Animal in the Animal Hall of Fame in 1969.

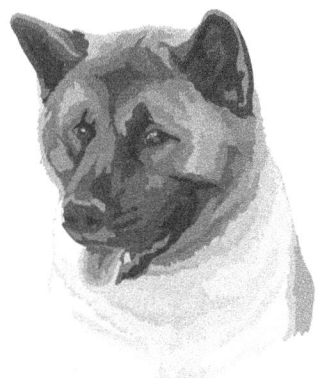

CHAPTER V:
A Reflection of God's Love

Genesis 1:31 – "God saw all that he had made, and it was very good."

GOD'S LOVE, CREATIVITY, AND UNIQUENESS

God's love is the foundation of all creation. Everything He has made---every tree, mountain, sunrise, and yes, even your dog--was crafted with intentionality and care. [Your Dog's Name] is not just an ordinary pet; they are a masterpiece of God's design, uniquely reflecting His creativity and love.

Have you ever noticed yourself smiling while watching [Your Dog's Name] do something quirky or endearing? Maybe you enjoy how they tilt their head when you talk to them, or how they race around the room with pure, uncontainable joy. These little behaviors are not random; they are glimpses of the beauty and creativity God poured into them.

God's love for us is evident in the timely arrival of specific animals in our lives. [Your Dog's Name] is a priceless gift, a vibrant representation of His love and compassion for you. Their presence reflects God's meticulous attention to detail and infinite creativity.

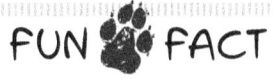

FUN FACT

Basenjis are the only dogs that do not bark. They yodel instead of barking.

In this chapter, we'll explore how [Your Dog's Name] reflects the beauty of God's love and uniqueness and how they reveal the nature of God Himself.

THE FOUR TYPES OF LOVE AS REFLECTED IN YOUR DOG

You may remember that in Chapter 2, we discussed the four types of love in the Greek language. Now, we will explore each of these in more depth, and how your dog demonstrates this kind of love towards you.

Agape (Unconditional Love):

Your dog loves you without conditions. Whether you have had a rough day or forgot their favorite treat, their love never wavers.

> Example: Think about how [Your Dog's Name] eagerly greets you at the door, no matter your day. This mirrors God's unconditional love for us.
>
> Scriptural Connection:
>
> *Romans 5:8 – "But God demonstrates his love for us in this: While we were still sinners, Christ died for us."*

Philia (Friendship or Brotherly Love):

Dogs are loyal companions, offering their friendship freely and without expectation.

> Example: Recall the moments when [Your Dog's Name] sits beside you, silently offering support as if to say, "I'm here, no matter what."
>
> Scriptural Connection:
>
> *John 15:13 – "Greater love has no one than this: to lay down one's life for one's friends."*

Storge (Familial Love):

Your dog is more than a pet; they are a cherished member of your family who brings warmth and joy into your home.

> Example: Consider how [Your Dog's Name] curls up by your side, making your house feel like a proper home.
>
> Scriptural Connection:

1 Timothy 5:8 – *"Anyone who does not provide for their relatives... has denied the faith."*

Eros (Delight in Beauty):

While traditionally romantic, Eros can also reflect our delight in the beauty of creation, including our dogs.

> Example: Consider how you marvel at [Your Dog's Name]'s soft fur, bright eyes, or joyful energy. These small details showcase God's creativity and love for beauty.
>
> Scriptural Connection:
>
> Genesis 1:31 – *"God saw all that he had made, and it was very good."*

GOD'S CREATIVITY IN YOUR DOG

God displays His creativity in countless ways, and your dog is a living example of His artistic touch. Here are four levels of creativity seen in [Your Dog's Name]:

> Spontaneous Creativity: When [Your Dog's Name] suddenly performs a funny trick or runs in joyful circles, it makes you smile. This spontaneity mirrors God's delight in surprising us with moments of joy.
>
> Deliberate Creativity: Consider how perfectly [Your Dog's Name] is designed, from their wagging tail to their keen instincts. Every feature, big and small, reflects God's intentional and thoughtful design.
>
> Cognitive Creativity: Consider the clever ways [Your Dog's Name] solves problems, like getting a treat from a challenging toy. This problem-solving ability is a reflection of God's wisdom and intelligence.
>
> Emotional Creativity: When [Your Dog's Name] senses your emotions and adjusts their behavior, offering comfort during sadness or playfulness during happiness, they reflect God's emotional depth and care for His children.

GOD'S LOVE THROUGH [YOUR DOG'S NAME]

Imagine if [Your Dog's Name] could see God from our lives. What would they think about God's love based on how you care for them? Use the following 2-3 pages to answer the questions below.

Reflect on how your actions—feeding, playing, and comforting [Your Dog's Name]--demonstrate God's love. Write specific examples showing how your care reflects His compassion and provision.

Consider how [Your Dog's Name] shows you God's love in return. Consider how their loyalty, comfort, and joy reflect God's character.

This activity helps you view your bond with [Your Dog's Name] as a two-way reflection of God's love and care for His creation.

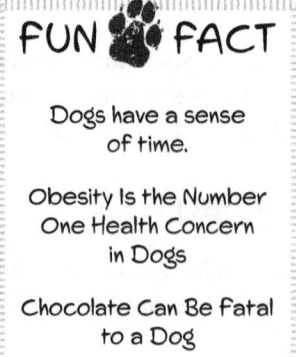

FUN FACT

Dogs have a sense of time.

Obesity Is the Number One Health Concern in Dogs

Chocolate Can Be Fatal to a Dog

— A REFLECTION OF GOD'S LOVE —

JOURNAL NOTES

JOURNAL NOTES

— A REFLECTION OF GOD'S LOVE —

JOURNAL NOTES

LET'S JOURNAL

Take the following 2-3 pages to answer the following questions below.

Unique Traits:

What are three unique things about [Your Dog's Name] that make them truly one-of-a-kind?

A Creative Moment:

Write about when [Your Dog's Name] brought creativity or joy into your day. How did that moment make you feel?

Seeing God's Creativity:

How do you see God's creativity reflected in [Your Dog's Name]'s behaviors, appearance, or personality?

Understanding God's Love:

In what ways has [Your Dog's Name] helped you better understand the depth and beauty of God's love?

A Personal Lesson:

If God designed [Your Dog's Name] specifically for you, what lessons do you think He wanted you to learn from them?

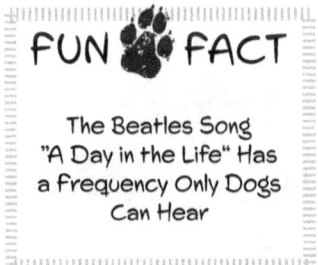

FUN FACT

The Beatles Song "A Day in the Life" Has a Frequency Only Dogs Can Hear

JOURNAL NOTES

JOURNAL NOTES

— A REFLECTION OF GOD'S LOVE —

JOURNAL NOTES

A POEM FOR [YOUR DOG'S NAME]

Genesis 1:31 – "God saw all that he had made, and it was very good."

Oh, [Your Dog's Name], a gift from above,

A living reflection of God's endless love.

Your wagging tail and joyful play,

Show me His care in every way.

Each bark, each nuzzle, so wonderfully made,

A glimpse of the beauty His hands have displayed.

In you, I see His creativity shine,

Oh, [Your Dog's Name], you're a blessing divine.

CLOSING THOUGHT

God's love, creativity, and purpose shine through in every aspect of your dog's existence. As you reflect on [Your Dog's Name], take note that they were crafted just for you, serving as a living reminder of God's goodness and compassion. Allow their distinctive quirks and characteristics to bring you nearer to the Creator, who has made both them and you in an extraordinary and flawless way.

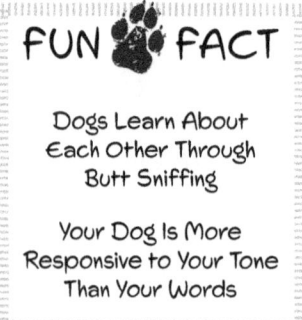

FUN 🐾 FACT

Dogs Learn About Each Other Through Butt Sniffing

Your Dog Is More Responsive to Your Tone Than Your Words

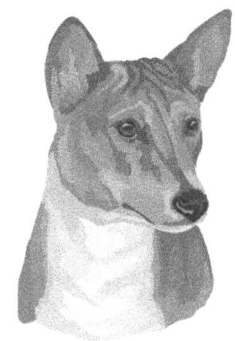

CHAPTER VI:
Gratitude for the Journey

Psalm 145:9 – "The Lord is good to all; he has compassion on all he has made."

TIME IS A GIFT

> "The greatest gift you can give someone is your time, because when you give your time, you are giving a portion of your life that you'll never get back."
> – Rick Warren

Every moment spent with our dogs is a treasured blessing from God. Life is short, and tomorrow is uncertain for everyone. This chapter encourages you to appreciate the time you have with [Your Dog's Name] – time filled with joy, lessons, and even challenges.

In His kindness, God brings companions like [Your Dog's Name] into our lives to enhance our experiences of love, joy, and care. Although our time together is not everlasting, it mirrors the beauty of God's eternal love for us. Savor each wag of the tail, every cuddle, and the quiet moments you share are tender reminders of God's compassion and the many blessings He gives us.

THE BEAUTY OF CHERISHING THE MOMENTS

Gratitude invites us to pause and recognize God's blessings, savoring the moments that might otherwise pass unnoticed. [Your Dog's Name] is one of those blessings uniquely created to share your journey. Every moment you spend together reflects God's love and goodness.

Examples of Cherished Moments with [Your Dog's Name]:

> **FUN FACT**
> The Saluki Is the Oldest Dog Breed

1. Morning Routines:

   The excitement and love [Your Dog's Name] shows when greeting you each morning mirrors God's mercies, which are new every day.

   Scripture Connection:

   Lamentations 3:22-23 – "His mercies are new every morning."

2. Playful Moments:

The joy of laughing at [Your Dog's Name]'s playful antics and quirky behaviors reminds us to embrace life's simple pleasures.

   Scripture Connection:

   Ecclesiastes 3:4 (NIV) – "A time to weep and a time to laugh, a time to mourn and a time to dance."

3. Quiet Companionship:

   Sitting in stillness with [Your Dog's Name] and feeling their warmth and presence reflects God's unwavering companionship.

   Scripture Connection:

   Psalm 46:10 (NIV) – "Be still, and know that I am God."

4. Challenges Together:

Even in challenging moments, such as training struggles or caring for [Your Dog's Name] during sickness, there are opportunities to grow in patience, faith, and resilience.

Scripture Connection:

James 1:2 - 4 (NIV) – *"Consider it pure joy, my brothers and sisters, whenever you face trials of many kinds, because you know that the testing of your faith produces perseverance. Let perseverance finish its work so that you may be mature and complete, not lacking anything."*

5. Goodbyes and Hellos:

When you return home, the enthusiastic welcome [Your Dog's Name] gives you reflects God's love for us when we draw closer to him.

Scripture Connection:

Luke 15:20 (NIV) – *"But while he was still a long way off, his father saw him and was filled with compassion for him; he ran to his son, threw his arms around him and kissed him."*

MOMENTS TO REMEMBER

Take a moment to answer the questions below over the next 2-3 pages. Recall your experiences with [Your Dog's Name], and note what thoughts and memories arise. I truly believe that if you reflect sufficiently, you'll discover plenty of memories, stories, and examples to draw from.

1. A First Correction:

    What was the first time you had to correct [Your Dog's Name]? How did they respond, and what did you learn from that moment?

2. Uncontrollable Laughter:

    Recall a time [Your Dog's Name] made you laugh so hard you could not stop. What happened, and how did it brighten your day?

3. A Comforting Presence:

    Consider a moment when [Your Dog's Name] comforted you during a difficult time. How did their presence make a difference?

4. A Memory to Treasure Forever:

    What is a recent memory with [Your Dog's Name] that you never want to forget?

5. A Reminder of Blessings:

    How have these moments with [Your Dog's Name] reminded you of God's blessings and care in your life?

FUN 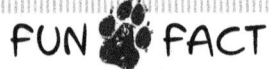 FACT

Toto's role in The Wizard of Oz was played by a female Cairn Terrier named Terry, and the Taco Bell dog is actually a female Chihuahua named Gidget

Dogs Were Domesticated Between 9,000 and 34,000 Years Ago

JOURNAL NOTES

JOURNAL NOTES

— GRATITUDE FOR THE JOURNEY —

JOURNAL NOTES

THE GRATITUDE GAME

Observe:

Sit with [Your Dog's Name] for 10 minutes and watch them. Notice their little quirks, such as how they wag their tail, tilt their head, stretch out for a nap, or do anything that makes them uniquely themselves.

Express Gratitude:

Write a sentence beginning with "I'm grateful for..." about each quirk.

> For example:
>
> "I'm grateful for how [Your Dog's Name] tilts their head when I talk to them, because it reminds me they are listening."
>
> "I'm grateful for [Your Dog's Name]'s snoring, because it means they feel safe and loved in my home."

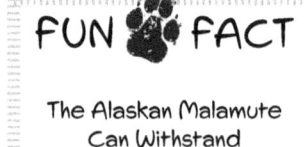

FUN FACT

The Alaskan Malamute Can Withstand Temperatures as Low as 50 Degrees Below Zero

Pray:

End the exercise with a simple prayer, thanking God for every unique detail that makes [Your Dog's Name] such a special part of your life.

LET'S JOURNAL

Take the following 2-3 pages to answer the questions below.

1. Memorable Moments:

> Think back on your time with [Your Dog's Name]. What moments stand out the most, and why are they so meaningful to you?

2. Cherished Qualities:

> List five things you cherish most about [Your Dog's Name]. How have these qualities enriched your life and brought you joy?

3. Lessons in Faith and Patience:

> Reflect on a challenging time you faced with [Your Dog's Name]. How did navigating that experience strengthen your faith or teach you patience?

4. Gratitude Overflow:

> Describe a moment when you felt overwhelming gratitude for [Your Dog's Name]. What triggered that feeling, and how did you express your thankfulness?

5. A Reflection of God's Goodness:

> How does [Your Dog's Name] remind you of God's compassion and care? Write about the ways their presence reflects His love in your life.

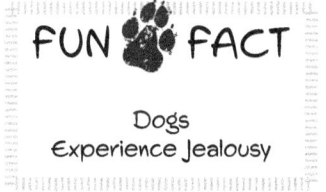

FUN FACT

Dogs Experience Jealousy

JOURNAL NOTES

JOURNAL NOTES

JOURNAL NOTES

THE TIME TO CHERISH EXERCISE

Take the following 2-3 pages to answer the questions below.

1. Three Words, One Dog:

   Describe [Your Dog's Name] in three words.

   Why did you choose those words, and how do they reflect who they are?

2. A Message from the Heart:

   Reflect on your time with [Your Dog's Name].

   What would you want to tell them if they could understand every word you said?

3. A Day to Relive:

   If you could go back and relive one day with [Your Dog's Name], which day would it be, and why is it so unique to you?

4. Their Perspective:

   What do you think [Your Dog's Name] cherishes most about you?

   How does this make you feel?

5. A Prayer of Gratitude:

   Write a heartfelt prayer thanking God for the gift of time and companionship with [Your Dog's Name]. Acknowledge the joy, lessons, and love they bring into your life.

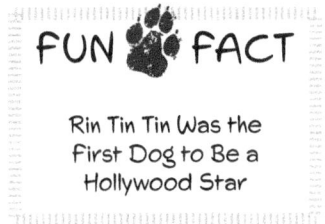

Rin Tin Tin Was the First Dog to Be a Hollywood Star

JOURNAL NOTES

— GRATITUDE FOR THE JOURNEY —

JOURNAL NOTES

JOURNAL NOTES

— GRATITUDE FOR THE JOURNEY —

GRATITUDE AS WORSHIP

Gratitude is a form of worship that honors the Giver of all good things. By cherishing [Your Dog's Name], you acknowledge God's blessings, compassion, and love in your life. Take a moment to reflect on this beautiful journey you've shared, and let every wag, bark, and cuddle remind you of God's endless care for you.

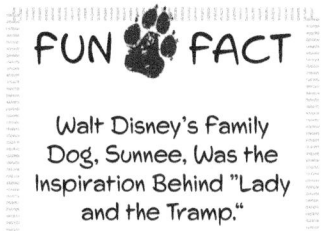

FUN FACT

Walt Disney's Family Dog, Sunnee, Was the Inspiration Behind "Lady and the Tramp."

— FUR-EVER FRIENDS —

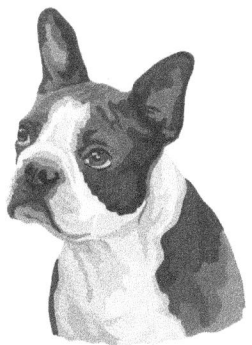

CHAPTER VII:
A Prayer for You and [Your Dog's Name]

Isaiah 43:20 – The animals honor me, the wild animals, because I provide water in the wilderness.

A HEART OF THANKFULNESS

Gratitude is one of the purest expressions of faith. By recognizing God's blessings and offering thanks, we draw closer to Him. Your dog, [Your Dog's Name], is one of those blessings, a living reminder of God's love, care, and provision.

God, in His perfect timing, brought [Fill in the blank] into your life. Each happy wag, playful bark, and peaceful moment together is more than happenstance; it is a reminder of His tender care and unwavering love for you.

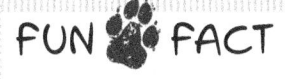

FUN FACT

Just Like Human Babies, Chihuahuas Are Born with soft spots

This chapter invites you to cultivate a heart of thankfulness, appreciating the unique joy and love [Your Dog's Name] brings into your life. Let their presence remind you of the countless ways God shows His goodness.

Thankfulness

The Bible reminds us often to live with a thankful heart, seeing God's blessings in every part of our lives:

Psalms 107:1 – "Give thanks to the Lord, for he is good; his love endures forever."

God's love is limitless, and your bond with [Your Dog's Name] reflects His goodness and care.

1 Thessalonians 5:18 – "Give thanks in all circumstances; for this is God's will for you in Christ Jesus."

Whether [Your Dog's Name] is playful, restful, or mischievous, there's always a reason to be grateful for their presence.

Isaiah 43:20 – "The animals honor me, the wild animals, because I provide water in the wilderness."

Just as God sustains every creature, He has provided for you and [Your Dog's Name], ensuring that His love nurtures your bond.

Examples of Thankfulness

Morning Gratitude

Each morning, as you feed or greet [Your Dog's Name], take a moment to thank God for another day with them. Reflect on the joy they bring to your life.

> Example: "Thank you, Lord, for [Your Dog's Name]'s wagging tail and the love they show me. Help me cherish this day with them."

Grateful Moments in the Day

When walking, playing, or simply sitting together, pause to reflect on how God has used [Your Dog's Name] to bring you closer to Him.

> Example: "Lord, I see your creativity in the way [Your Dog's Name] plays and your love in the comfort they bring me."

— A PRAYER FOR YOU AND [YOUR DOG'S NAME] —

End-of-Day Reflection

Before bed, thank God for the day's moments with [Your Dog's Name], whether a simple cuddle or a silly adventure.

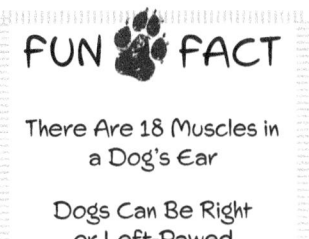

FUN FACT

There Are 18 Muscles in a Dog's Ear

Dogs Can Be Right or Left-Pawed

Example: "Father, thank you for [Your Dog's Name]'s companionship today. They are a reminder of your faithfulness and love."

WHAT WOULD [YOUR DOG'S NAME] THANK YOU FOR?

Take the following 2-3 pages to answer the questions below.

Imagine Your Dog Could Speak:

Close your eyes and picture [Your Dog's Name] sitting before you, ready to express their gratitude. What do you think they'd say? Would it be for the food you provide, the belly rubs, or the time you spend together?

Create a Gratitude List:

- List specific things you do for [Your Dog's Name], big and small, that show your love and care. Examples might include:
- Feeding them their favorite meals.
- Going on walks, even when you're tired.
- Offering comfort during thunderstorms.
- Playing their favorite game or giving them treats.

Draw Parallels to God's Care:

- Reflect on how these acts of care mirror God's provision in your life. For example:
- Just as you provide food and water for your dog, God provides for your physical needs.

- Your comforting of [Your Dog's Name] during scary moments reflects God's calming presence in your life.

Write a Note of Gratitude:

End this exercise by writing a short note of thanks to God, inspired by how you care for [Your Dog's Name]. For instance:

- "Thank You, Lord, for entrusting me with [Your Dog's Name]. I've learned about Your love, provision, and care through them. Help me to continue reflecting Your goodness in how I care for them."

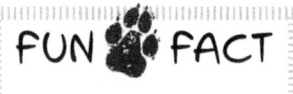

FUN FACT

Storm noises can be painful for dogs' ears, and they might also experience discomfort from static electricity. If your dog becomes anxious during a thunderstorm, offer comfort and understanding.

St. Bernards are used as search and rescue dogs.

— A PRAYER FOR YOU AND [YOUR DOG'S NAME] —

JOURNAL NOTES

JOURNAL NOTES

— A PRAYER FOR YOU AND [YOUR DOG'S NAME] —

JOURNAL NOTES

— FUR-EVER FRIENDS —

LET'S JOURNAL

Use the following 2-3 pages to answer the questions below.

1. Three Things You're Thankful For

Take a moment to list three specific things about [Your Dog's Name] that bring you the most joy. Is it their playful nature, comforting presence, or perhaps the way they greet you with endless enthusiasm? Reflect on why these qualities mean so much to you.

2. Lessons of Gratitude and Love

How has God used [Your Dog's Name] to reveal lessons about gratitude and love? Perhaps their unconditional devotion has taught you about God's unwavering care, or their patience has mirrored God's grace.

3. A Moment to Remember

Recall a moment when [Your Dog's Name] gave you profound joy or comfort. Was it when they curled up next to you during a time you needed a friend, or the simple happiness of sharing a fun adventure? Describe that experience in your own words and take a moment to cherish it.

4. Showing Gratitude Every Day

How can you express daily thankfulness to God for the blessing of [Your Dog's Name]? Maybe through prayer, cherishing quiet moments with your dog, or simply pausing to appreciate your bond.

5. One Word to Describe Your Relationship

If you had to sum up your connection with [Your Dog's Name] in a single word, what would it be? Love? Loyalty? Joy? Why does this word resonate so profoundly with your bond?

FUN FACT

Dogs can hear 40 to 60,000 Hz, while humans can only hear 20 Hz to 20,000 Hz.

A dog's whiskers are full of nerves and act as multifunctional sensory tools. They help them move around and maneuver, especially in low-visibility settings.

— A PRAYER FOR YOU AND [YOUR DOG'S NAME] —

JOURNAL NOTES

JOURNAL NOTES

— A PRAYER FOR YOU AND [YOUR DOG'S NAME] —

JOURNAL NOTES

A SPECIAL PRAYER FOR [YOUR DOG'S NAME]

Rejoice always, pray continually, give thanks in all circumstances; for this is God's will for you in Christ Jesus. – 1 Thessalonians 5:16-18 16

"Dear Heavenly Father,

Thank you for blessing [Your Dog's Name]. They reflect your love, creativity, and provision in my life. Thank you for their wagging tail, playful spirit, and comfort.

"Help me to cherish every moment with [Your Dog's Name], knowing that each day is a gift from You. Teach me to love them well, as you love all of your creation.

"I pray for [Your Dog's Name]'s health and happiness. May they always feel safe, loved, and cared for. Thank you for our bond and the lessons they teach me about joy, patience, and unconditional love.

"In Jesus' name, Amen."

ENCOURAGEMENT TO CREATE YOUR PRAYER

I want to encourage you to create your prayer(s) of gratitude for [Your Dog's Name]. This could include thanking God for specific moments, asking for continued blessings, and expressing their love for their dog.

These four principles have guided me in receiving answers to my prayers, and I wish to share them with you:

1. Trust in the One you are praying to

2. Pray in alignment with God's word

3. Have faith that your prayer is answered the moment you pray

4. Anticipate the answer to your prayer, knowing you are simply awaiting its manifestation or outcome.

— A PRAYER FOR YOU AND [YOUR DOG'S NAME] —

JOURNAL NOTES

JOURNAL NOTES

— A PRAYER FOR YOU AND [YOUR DOG'S NAME] —

TIMELINE OF THANKFULNESS

Take a moment to pause and reflect on where you are today with [Your Dog's Name]. How has your bond changed since the day you first met? Think about the trust that has been built, the adventures you've shared, and the challenges you've faced together. Has your dog's presence shaped the way you see love, loyalty, or even life itself? Write about the journey, both the big moments and the small, everyday ones that have strengthened your connection.

This activity allows you to celebrate and cherish your journey together while thanking God for the gift of [Your Dog's Name].

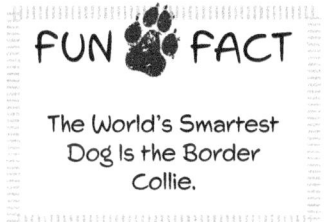

FUN FACT

The World's Smartest Dog is the Border Collie.

JOURNAL NOTES

— A PRAYER FOR YOU AND [YOUR DOG'S NAME] —

JOURNAL NOTES

JOURNAL NOTES

CLOSING THOUGHT: GRATITUDE AS WORSHIP

Gratitude is more than just an emotion; it is a form of worship. By thanking God for [Your Dog's Name], you acknowledge His goodness and the thoughtful ways He cares for you. Each moment spent with [Your Dog's Name], whether a wagging tail, a playful bark, or a quiet cuddle, is a reminder of God's constant love and provision.

Make gratitude a daily practice to connect more deeply with the Creator, who thoughtfully brought [Your Dog's Name] into your life. May your heart be filled with appreciation for the joy and blessings they bring to your world as you progress on this journey.

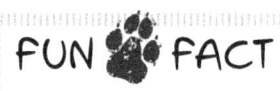

Kids who read to real animals showed better social skills, more sharing, cooperation, and volunteering, and fewer behavioral problems.

— FUR-EVER FRIENDS —

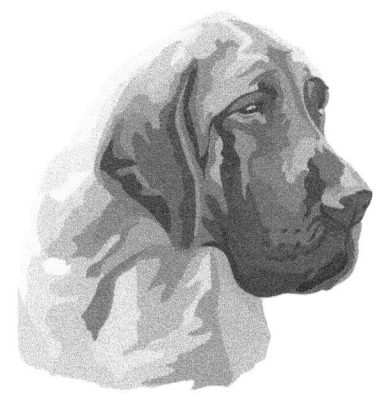

CHAPTER VIII:

The Power of Your Words

"Death and life are in the power of the tongue, and those who love it and indulge in it will eat its fruit and bear the consequences of their words."
– Proverbs 18:21

YOUR WORDS HAVE POWER, SO WATCH WHAT YOU SAY!

Key Scriptures:

Proverbs 15:4 – *"The soothing tongue is a tree of life, but a perverse tongue crushes the spirit."*

Colossians 4:6 – *"Let your conversation be always full of grace, seasoned with salt, so that you may know how to answer everyone."*

Proverbs 18:21 – *"The tongue has the power of life and death, and those who love it will eat its fruit."*

Ephesians 4:29 – *"Do not let any unwholesome talk come out of your mouths, but only what helps build others up according to their needs, that it may benefit those who listen."*

THE POWER OF YOUR WORDS

Have you ever noticed how your dog reacts to your voice? The tone you use, the words you choose, and the emotions behind them significantly impact your dog. Dogs are incredibly intuitive beings, finely attuned to the energy we emit. When we speak with encouragement and kindness, they thrive. However, when our words are harsh or filled with negativity, it can dampen their spirits in ways we may not fully grasp.

The Bible consistently highlights the tremendous influence of our words. Proverbs 18:21 Notes, "The tongue has the power of life and death, and those who love it will eat its fruit." This principle applies to our interactions with others and encompasses God's creation, including your cherished dog. Your dog, [Your Dog's Name], doesn't merely hear what you say; they perceive the emotions underlying your words. Just as God listens to and engages with us during prayer, your dog intuitively understands the feelings behind your words and voice.

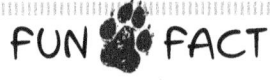

Many dogs serve as guide dogs for people who are blind, assistance dogs for calming their owners, and search and rescue dogs that aid in saving lives.

Words are more than mere sounds; they embody intention, energy, and influence. When you say, "good dog," with heartfelt warmth, your dog understands that it has performed well and is cherished. On the other hand, negative words can bewilder or harm them, especially when spoken in anger. Such instances impart a significant lesson about our duty to choose words thoughtfully and kindly.

This chapter examines the impact of your words on your dog's well-being and behavior, the importance of speaking positively to them, and how this practice aligns with God's call to be compassionate stewards of His creation. By recognizing the link between our words and their effects, we can strengthen our bond with our dogs and enrich our relationship with God, who has entrusted us with these beloved companions' care.

REFLECTIONS FOR A FRIEND

Think about a time when your words immediately impacted your dog. How did they react, and what did it teach you about their sensitivity?

How does how you speak to your dog reflect your understanding of God's call to speak with love and grace?

Proverbs 15:4 "The soothing tongue is a tree of life, but a perverse tongue crushes the spirit." Just as our kind words can uplift those around us, they can nurture and encourage our dogs.

Ephesians 4:29: "Do not let any unwholesome talk come out of your mouths, but only what helps build others up according to their needs."

This verse reminds us that our speech should be constructive, even when addressing our pets, who look to us for guidance and affection.

Actionable Takeaways

Speak Life Daily: Begin each day by speaking words of love and encouragement to [Your Dog's Name]. For example, "Good morning, [Your Dog's Name]! I'm so glad you're here with me."

Pause Before You Speak: If you are feeling frustrated, take a moment to breathe before addressing your dog. Remember, they are trying their best to understand you.

Use Positive Reinforcement: Celebrate their good behavior with affirming words and a warm tone. It strengthens your bond and encourages them to keep trying.

Your dog is a gift from God, a reminder of His love and care. Just as He speaks life over us through His Word, we can do the same for our furry companions. Let your words be a source of comfort, encouragement, and joy for [Your Dog's Name], reflecting the heart of a loving Creator.

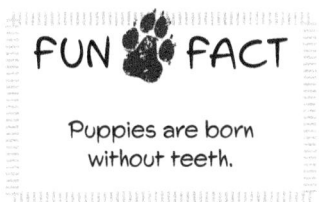

FUN FACT

Puppies are born without teeth.

EXPLAINING THE SCRIPTURES

Proverbs 15:4 – "The soothing tongue is a tree of life, but a perverse tongue crushes the spirit."

This scripture reminds us that kind, gentle words bring life, healing, and comfort, while harsh words can harm the spirit.

Example: Think about the times you've spoken softly to [Your Dog's Name] when they were scared, such as during a thunderstorm. Your soothing tone likely calmed them and reassured them of your presence. Contrast that with times you may have spoken harshly or yelled; they likely reacted with fear or sadness.

Colossians 4:6 – "Let your conversation be always full of grace, seasoned with salt."

This verse teaches us to speak gracefully and intentionally, ensuring our words uplift and benefit others, including our dogs.

Example: When training your dog, try praising what they do right instead of focusing on what they do wrong. Positive reinforcement not only encourages better behavior but also strengthens your bond.

Proverbs 18:21 – "The tongue has the power of life and death."

Our words plant seeds that grow into life or death. Speaking kindly to [Your Dog's Name] plants seeds of trust, love, and joy, while negative words can sow fear or insecurity.

Example: If you enthusiastically say, "good dog!", it lifts their spirits. However, repeatedly calling them "bad dogs" can discourage them and negatively affect their behavior.

Ephesians 4:29 – "Do not let any unwholesome talk come out of your mouths."

This verse reminds us to speak only what helps build others up, ensuring our words benefit those who hear them.

Example: Replace phrases like "You're so annoying" with affirmations like "You're so special to me." It changes the atmosphere of your relationship with [Your Dog's Name].

PRACTICAL EXERCISES

The Daily Blessing:

Start each day by speaking a blessing over [Your Dog's Name]. Say something like: "You are loved, you are cherished, and you are a gift from God. Thank you for bringing joy to my life." Reflect on how this daily habit uplifts your dog and reminds you of God's blessings.

Positive Word Swap:

> Make a list of phrases you might say in frustration (e.g., "You're so bad!"). Next to each phrase, write a positive alternative (e.g., "Let's try again, buddy!"), practice using the positive options daily.

Speak Scripture Over Your Dog:

> Choose a scripture like Proverbs 15:4 or Psalm 145:9 and say it aloud to your dog each day. For example: "The Lord is good to all, including you, [Your Dog's Name]. He has compassion on all He has made, including you!"

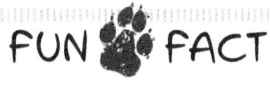

FUN FACT

Puppies spend 15-20 hours a day sleeping

Newborn puppies have heat sensors in their noses to help find their mother while their eyes and ears are closed.

Puppies grow to half their body weight in the first 4-5 months.

The Thankful Tone Check:

> Throughout the day, pause to reflect on your tone when speaking to [Your Dog's Name]. If it's harsh or impatient, take a moment to rest and speak with kindness instead.

Name Their Strengths:

> Each evening, say aloud three things you love or appreciate about [Your Dog's Name]. This reinforces positive interactions and

Gratitude.

SPEAKING LIFE TO [YOUR DOG'S NAME]

Take the following 2-3 pages to answer the questions below.

Kindness vs. Harshness: How do you think [Your Dog's Name] feels when you speak to them kindly versus harshly? Reflect on specific moments and consider how you can be more intentional in speaking gently.

Daily Affirmations: List three affirmations or kind phrases you can say to [Your Dog's Name] daily. For example, "You're such a good dog," "I love having you in my life," or "Thank you for being my friend." How do these words positively impact their behavior and your bond?

Reflecting on Negativity: Think about a time when you may have said something negative or used a harsh tone with [Your Dog's Name]. How did they respond? What can you learn from that moment, and how can you approach similar situations gracefully and patiently?

God's Example: God speaks to us with love, patience, and kindness, even when we make mistakes. How can you reflect this divine example in communicating with [Your Dog's Name]?

A Prayer for Words of Life: Write a prayer asking God to guide your words so they bring life and encouragement not just to [Your Dog's Name] but to everyone you encounter. Ask for wisdom to see how your words impact others and to use them to glorify Him.

JOURNAL NOTES

JOURNAL NOTES

JOURNAL NOTES

ENCOURAGEMENT TO SPEAK LIFE

Words are seeds; what you say to [Your Dog's Name] truly matters. Your dog may not comprehend every word, but they can perceive the tone, energy, and emotions behind your words. Speak life, love, and encouragement over them daily, just as God imparts life to you through His Word. God's Word is life, not only to you but to every living being. Therefore, ensure your language promotes life for people, creation, situations, challenges, and every creature. Remember Proverbs 18:21 and Matthew 7:12!

CLOSING THOUGHT

Your words can significantly enhance your bond with [Your Dog's Name]. By speaking positively, you not only honor God but also uplift your dog while creating a loving and grateful environment. Start today by sharing your experiences, planting seeds of kindness, and watching as your relationship with [Your Dog's Name] deepens and grows

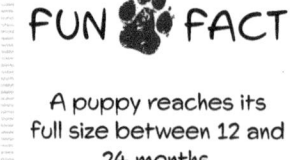

FUN FACT

A puppy reaches its full size between 12 and 24 months.

affectionately. As you express your wishes for you and your dog, keep **Mark 11:23-24** in mind. Additionally, remember that others also have pets and may not grasp the insights from this book. I urge you to extend your knowledge to them, linking them to God's word and its significance for their pets. It is essential for them to recognize and honor Him, just as we do, given that He has blessed them with a wonderful furry friend.

GAME: "WORDS OF LIFE SCAVENGER HUNT"

Objective: Strengthen your bond with your dog through positive communication while creating a fun and enriching activity.

What You'll Need:

- Your dog's favorite treats or toys.
- A few index cards or pieces of paper.
- A marker or pen.

Setup

Write down five positive affirmations or kind phrases on the index cards. For example:

- "You are loved, [Your Dog's Name]!"
- "You are a blessing to me!"
- "You bring joy into my life every day!"
- "You are fearfully and wonderfully made!"
- "You are the best friend I could ever ask for!"

Hide the cards around your home or yard in places your dog can safely explore.

Pair each card with a small treat or toy to make it a rewarding discovery for your dog.

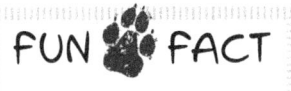

FUN FACT

A dog's foot, often called a "paw," consists of pads, claws, and other structures that help with various functions.

How to Play

Begin the hunt by saying, "Let's find some love!" or "Let's go on a treasure hunt!" Encourage your dog to search for the hidden cards using playful tones and gestures.

When your dog finds a card, read the affirmation aloud to it excitedly and lovingly. Then, celebrate with claps, belly rubs, or a happy "Good dog!" to reinforce the positivity. Give them a treat or toy as a reward for finding the card.

Reflection: After the game, sit down with your dog and reflect on the affirmations you shared. Thank God for the joy your dog brings and for the ability to speak life and love into their world

Why This Works

For Your Dog:

> The scavenger hunt is a mentally stimulating activity that engages their senses and builds positive associations with your words.

For You:

It reinforces the habit of speaking life and appreciating your dog's presence while deepening your connection with them.

For Your Bond:

This game fosters trust and love, strengthening the bond between you and your dog in a fun and uplifting way.

Fun Fact: Dogs typically live 8 to 15 years, but the oldest recorded dog, Bluey, lived 29 years and 5 months. Born in Australia in 1910, he worked with cattle and sheep for nearly two decades. In human years, that's over 200 years!

A FEW EXERCISES TO TRY ON YOUR OWN

Reflection Collage:

Gather pictures, drawings, or words representing your journey with [Your Dog's Name].

Arrange them into a visual collage that you can keep as a reminder of your bond and God's blessings.

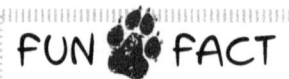

FUN FACT

The bottom of a dog's paw has thick, cushioned pads that provide protection and traction. These pads also contain sweat glands that help regulate body temperature.

Dogs have a membrane called the tapetum lucidum, enabling them to see in the dark. Thus, their beautiful blue or chestnut eyes appear green or diluted in dim light.

Thanksgiving Walk:

Take [Your Dog's Name] for a walk. With each step, thank God for something specific about your dog, their quirks, their love, or the lessons they've taught you.

Prayer of Dedication:

Spend time writing a prayer, dedicating your bond with [Your Dog's Name] to God. Thank Him for the joy, the challenges, and the companionship they bring into your life.

LET'S JOURNAL

Take the following 2-3 pages to answer the questions below.

1. Through Their Eyes

Imagine a day in your life from [Fill in the blank]'s perspective.

> How might they see you, your habits, your moods, and your love for them? What would they notice most about your heart?

2. Spiritual Footprints

Think of three moments when [Fill in the blank] unknowingly modeled a truth about God's character, like patience, forgiveness, or unconditional love.

> How have those moments shaped your understanding of Him?

3. Sacred Encounters

Recall a time when you felt God speaking to you through something [Fill in the blank] did, whether it was in their comfort, their joy, or even their stubbornness.

> What message do you think God was sending in that moment?

4. Gratitude as a Lifestyle

Instead of a single act of thanks, picture what it would look like if every day with [Your Dog's Name] became an act of worship.

> How might you live differently to honor both God and this gift He's given you?

5. Eternal Companionship

If God gave you a few moments in heaven to speak to [Fill in the blank], knowing they could fully understand, what would you say to them about your journey together on earth and the role they played in your faith story?

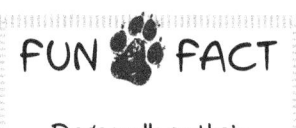

FUN FACT

Dogs walk on their toes, a stance known as digitigrade, in which they bear weight on their digits or toe bones rather than on the entire foot.

JOURNAL NOTES

JOURNAL NOTES

JOURNAL NOTES

GRATITUDE JAR

Create a "Gratitude Jar" for [Your Dog's Name].

Write down one thing you're thankful for about them daily and place it in the jar.

Over time, watch the jar fill up with reminders of God's goodness and your dog's impact on your life.

FROM MY HEART TO YOURS AND [YOUR DOG'S NAME]

Dear Friend,

As you close this book, thank you for your time, for opening your heart, for engaging with these reflections, and for embracing the beautiful bond you share with [Your Dog's Name]. I hope this journey has offered you a fresh perspective on your beloved companion and the infinite love and care our Creator has for you.

Caring for [Your Dog's Name] is no small task. You have chosen to nurture and cherish one of God's voiceless creations, offering them kindness, patience, and unconditional love. This is a sacred responsibility, and I thank God for the heart you have for your dog. Through your care, you reflect God's compassion and grace in ways that make the world a little brighter.

Your time with [Your Dog's Name] is a precious blessing. Whether it is a wagging tail that greets you at the end of a long day, a playful bark that lifts your spirits, or a quiet moment of companionship, these interactions reflect God's goodness and creativity. Each moment together is a gift to be cherished. I pray that you and [Your Dog's Name] continue to create countless joyful memories filled with love, laughter, and gratitude.

As you move forward, I encourage you to remain connected to God. Thank Him daily for the blessings in your life, trust Him with the journey ahead (Jeremiah 29:11), and lean on Him in both joyous and challenging times. Remember that the bond you share with [Your Dog's Name] reminds you of God's unwavering love and faithfulness.

Stay blessed, stay grateful, and know that you are deeply loved by your dog and the God who made you both.

With heartfelt gratitude,

Sean

ENCOURAGEMENT TO CONTINUE THE JOURNEY

As we conclude our journey through this book, I encourage you to maintain the connection between the blessings God has bestowed upon you through your furry companion and His love for you. If I were to encapsulate this book in a single word, it would be "relationship." That is what God desires with each one of us: a personal connection. This book aims to provide you with a fresh lens through which to appreciate and love your furry friend. I feel honored to share my perspective on how our furry companions enhance our lives. Now, as you embark on this new journey with your animal companion, [Your Dog's Name], let it be a path filled with love, lessons, and faith. Keep close the reminders of God's love, creativity, and care. Cherish the joy and gratitude from the insights you have recorded, motivating you to love deeply, live fully, and trust God wholeheartedly in every moment spent with [Your Dog's Name].

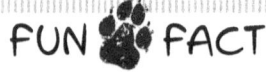

Dog paws contain many sensory receptors, making them sensitive to touch, pressure, and temperature. This sensitivity aids their navigation and interaction with the environment.

Dog paw shapes and sizes can vary based on the breed, size, and individual characteristics. Some breeds have webbed paws, which aid in swimming.

THANK YOU

Dear Friend,

Thank you for reading *Fur-Ever Friends: A Journey with Your Sacred Companion.* Your decision to explore this book, which delves into the deep connections between God's love, your dog's steadfast loyalty, and your personal spiritual journey, means more to me than I can articulate. I consider it a privilege to share this heartfelt project with you, and I sincerely appreciate your support.

This book originates from a wish to ignite a movement and change in our perception and treatment of our furry friends. Dogs are not just responsibilities we accept; they are precious gifts given to us, representing God's unwavering love and faithfulness. Their companionship allows us to witness aspects of God's care, patience, and joy. I hope this book inspires a fresh viewpoint, motivating you to value and honor the privilege of being chosen to be a dog owner.

Through reading *Fur-Ever Friends,* I also aim to shed light on the numerous dogs in shelters that require loving homes. By deepening our appreciation for the unique bond between humans and dogs, we can foster empathy and encourage action, ensuring these animals receive the love and companionship they deserve. Whether you already have a dog, wish to adopt one, or simply appreciate these amazing beings, you belong to a community that can drive positive change.

Your feedback is invaluable to me. I would love to hear how this book has impacted you, whether it blessed, encouraged, or even fell short of your expectations. Honest insights from readers like you help me grow and better serve this incredible community of dog lovers. Please email me at **fur-everblessed@mail.com** to share your thoughts and experiences.

This journey extends far beyond the book. I am excited to share that we are introducing new initiatives aimed at fostering deeper connections and engagement within our community. This will include a YouTube channel, a dedicated app, and additional resources designed to inspire and uplift. By staying connected, you will be among the first to learn about these thrilling developments. Together, we can continue to spark humanity, kindness, and love, celebrating our diversity while embracing the unique gifts and creativity that God has given us.

In an increasingly isolated world, it is essential to concentrate on what really counts: loving, serving, and supporting each other, much like we do for our beloved pets. With God as the ultimate Alpha of our human pack, we can foster a community centered on love, compassion, unity, and grace.

Again, thank you for your time, support, and heart for this mission. I look forward to hearing from you and continuing this journey together.

With gratitude and blessings,

Sean James
Author, *Fur-Ever Friends: A Journey with Your Sacred Companion*

Email: fureverblessed7@gmail.com

TikTok: fureverblessed

Instagram: fureverblessed1

SCRIPTURAL REFERENCES

1 Kings 17:4-6
Romans 12:10 Proverbs 12:10
Psalms 36:6
Numbers 22:21-33
Matthew 6:34
Psalm 145:9
Ephesians 2:8-9
Genesis 7:1-16
Psalm 139:14
Isaiah 43:20
Psalms 34:18
Isaiah 41:10
Romans 5:8
Psalm 104:24 1

Thessalonians 5:16-18
Isaiah 54:10
John 15:13
eremiah 29:11
Philippians 4:13
Ecclesiastes 3:1 1
Timothy 5:8
Joshua 1:5
Lamentations 3:22-23
Genesis 1:31
Proverbs 18:21
Philippians 4:19
Psalm 107:1
Proverbs 15:4
Romans 8:38-39 1

Thessalonians 5:18
Colossians 4:6
Galatians 6:2
James 1:17
Ephesians 4:29
Psalm 86:15
Psalm 36:6
Matthew 7:12
Proverbs 3:5
1 John 4:19
Mark 11:23-241
John 4:8
Joshua 1:9
Hebrews 4:16

GOD'S LOVE FOR YOU AND YOUR DOG

Dear Friend,

Here are a few additional reminders of God's love for you. Indeed, they are meant specifically for you as you read this book, connecting to the unique bond you share with your furry companion. I hope and pray they resonate with you.

1. God's Love is Unfailing

    Paraphrased Verse:

    "God's love never ends, and He is always kind." (Lamentations 3:22-23)

    Promise: God's love and kindness are new every morning, no matter what happens.

2. God Loves You So Much He Gave His Son

    Paraphrased Verse:

    "God loved the world so much that He sent His only Son, so everyone who believes in Him can have life forever." (John 3:16)

    Promise: God loves you enough to give you eternal life through Jesus.

3. God's Love is Perfect.

    Paraphrased Verse:

    "God loves you perfectly, and His love makes you brave." (1 John 4:18)

    Promise: You don't need to be afraid because God's love is more prominent than fear.

4. God Knows and Loves You Personally

    Paraphrased Verse:

    "God made you and knows everything about you. His thoughts about you are precious!" (Psalm 139:13-14, 17)

    Promise: God created you wonderfully and thinks about you all the time.

5. God Will Never Stop Loving You.

    Paraphrased Verse:

    "Nothing can take God's love away from you." (Romans 8:38-39)

    Promise: No matter what happens, God's love for you will never change.

6. God Loves You Just as You Are ·

    Paraphrased Verse:

    "Even before you loved Him, God showed His love by sending Jesus to save you." (Romans 5:8)

    Promise: God loves you so much that He reached out to you first.

— SCRIPTURE REFERENCES —

7. God's Love is Forever.

    Paraphrased Verse:

    "God's love lasts forever." (Psalm 136:26)

    Promise: God's love does not run out or fade away.

8. God's Love Brings Comfort.

    Paraphrased Verse:

    "When you're sad, God's love can make your heart happy again." (Psalm 34:18)

    Promise: God is close to you when you are feeling brokenhearted.

9. God's Love Helps You Be Strong.

    Paraphrased Verse:

    "With God's love, you can be strong and brave." (Deuteronomy 31:6)

    Promise: God will never leave you alone; His love gives you courage.

10. God's Love Fills Your Heart.

    Paraphrased Verse:

    "God pours His love into your heart through His Spirit." (Romans 5:5)

    Promise: God's love fills you up so you can share it with others.

— FUR-EVER FRIENDS —

REFERENCES

1. Caulfield, J. (2023, December 1). *How to Cite the Bible in APA Style | Format & Examples*. Scribbr. Retrieved December 30, 2024, from https://www.scribbr.com/apa-examples/bible/

2. Bible Gateway.com: A searchable online Bible available in over 150 versions and 50 languages. (n.d.). https://biblegateway.com/

3. Read the Bible online: access a free Bible on your phone, tablet, or computer. | *The Bible App* | Bible.com. (n.d.). YouVersion | The Bible App |Bible.com. https://bible.com/

4. U.S. pet ownership statistics. (n.d.). *American Veterinary Medical Association*. https://www.avma.org/resources-tools/reports-statistics/us-pet-ownership-statistics

5. Kriss, R. (2024, April 17). "Most popular dog breeds." *American Kennel Club*. https://www.akc.org/most-popular-breeds/

6. Habri. (2024, May 2). "How pets impact our mental health." *HABRI*. https://habri.org/blog/how-pets-impact-our-mental-health/

7. "Pets and mental health." (n.d.). *Mental Health Foundation*. https://www.mentalhealth.org.uk/explore-mental-health/a-z-topics/pets-and-mental- health

8. "Health benefits of pet ownership." (2024). *Veterinary Medical Center*. https://vmc.vet.osu.edu/resources/health-benefits-pet-ownership

9. Manis, E. (2024, April 17). "New study sheds light on the positive and negative impacts of dog ownership on psychological wellbeing." *PsyPost - Psychology News*. https://www.psypost.org/new-study-sheds-light-on-the-positive-and-negative-impacts-of-dog-ownership-on-psychologicalwellbeing/

10. "The power of pets." (2024, June 17). NIH *News in Health*. https://newsinhealth.nih.gov/2018/02/power-pets

11. Staff, A. (2023, August 2). "30 Fun and fascinating dog facts." *American Kennel Club.* https://www.akc.org/expert-advice/lifestyle/dog-facts/

12. Cosgrove, N. (2024, December 12). "50 fun facts about dogs you will love to know." *Dogster.* https://www.dogster.com/lifestyle/fun-dog-facts

13. "30 amazing facts about dogs that will blow your mind"| *Purina.* (n.d.). https://www.purina.co.uk/articles/dogs/behaviour/common- questions/amazing-dog-facts

14. Giordano, R. (2024, July 23). "35 Famous Dogs on TV & Movies (With Pictures)." *PangoVet.* https://pangovet.com/pet-lifestyle/dogs/famous-dogs- on-tv-movies/

15. Bogage, J. (2022, January 7). "Americans adopt millions of dogs during a pandemic. Now what do we do with them?" *Washington Post* https://www.washingtonpost.com/business/2022/01/07/covid-dogs-return-to-work/

16. "Dog Facts for Kids!" | *National Geographic Kids.* https://www.natgeokids.com/uk/discover/animals/general-animals/dog-facts/

17. Jan. (2020, July 14). "20 interesting facts about puppies." *Pawfect Surprise.* https://www.pawfectsurprise.com/post/20-interesting-facts-about- puppies

18. "10 Things You Never Knew about your dog "- The Dog Blog | *Expert advice for pet parents.* (n.d.). Bil-Jac. https://www.bil-jac.com/the-dog- blog/posts/10-things-you-never-knew-about-your-dog/

19. K9anytime. (2023, October 12). "11 Dog Feet Facts." *k9anytime.* https://www.k9anytime.com/single-post/11-dog-feet-facts

20. Staff, B. I. (2022, April 17). "8 stories of hero dogs saving human lives" [Video]. *Be Inspired.* https://beinspired.global/8-stories-of-hero-dogs- saving-human-lives/

21. Care, P. V. (n.d.). "23 Amazing facts about dogs you probably didn't know." *4 Paws Veterinary Care.* https://www.4pawsanimal.com/services/dogs/blog/23-amazing-facts-about-dogs-you-probably-didnt-know

22. The MSPCA-Angell. (2017, March 15). "Interesting Facts about dogs" *MSPCA-Angell.* MSPCA-Angell. https://www.mspca.org/pet_resources/interesting-facts-about-dogs/

ABOUT SEAN JAMES

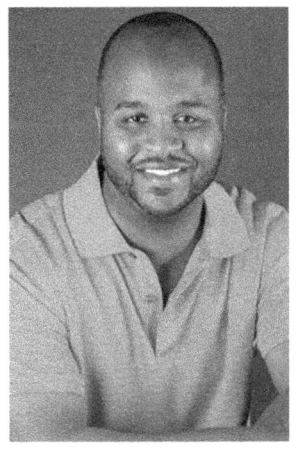

Born and raised in Illinois, I grew up in a Christian household where my amazing mother taught me that keeping God first is the foundation of life. That faith carried me through my journey from studying communications in college to packing my bags and heading out to Los Angeles in 2004, all fueled by a dream to act.

Once I landed in L.A., I found myself on set and quickly had a shift in perspective. I realized I didn't just want to be in front of the camera as an actor, essentially an employee, but to be behind the scenes as the owner, the creator of meaningful stories. More importantly, God placed a calling on my heart to change the narrative of the messages we share with kids and families. As we know, with God, all things are possible.

That's how the vision for Furever Blessed (the company) was born, and now my first book, Furever Friends, has been penned and has come to fruition, but that's just one piece of a bigger puzzle. My goal? To uplift those battling depression, isolation, or loneliness by showing them that God's love is often reflected in the companionship of a dog.

Ultimately, I'm just a person with a small but beloved family, a passion for sharing God's truth, and a mission to inspire through edifying faith-driven stories. I believe we can all make the world a little brighter, one wagging tail and one heartfelt story at a time.

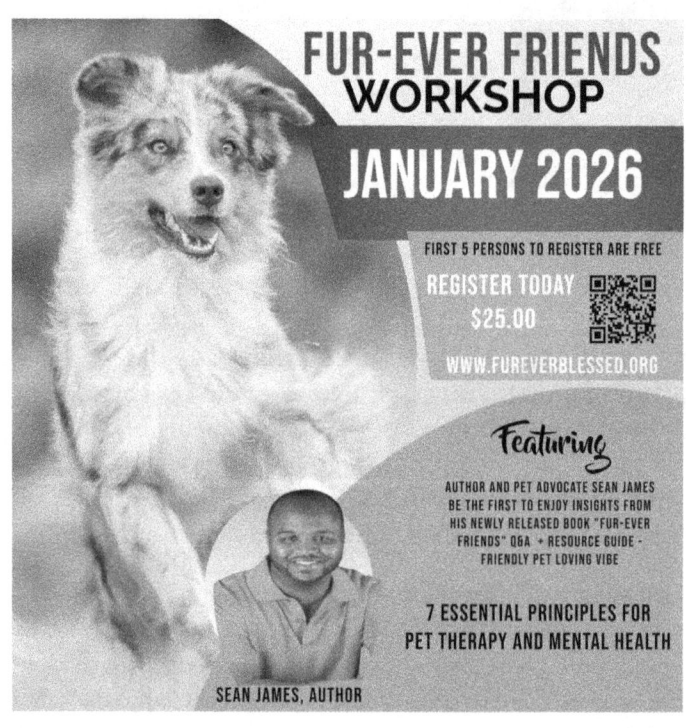

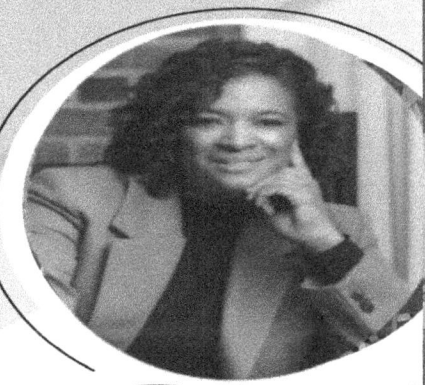

— FUR-EVER FRIENDS —

www.ingramcontent.com/pod-product-compliance
Lightning Source LLC
Chambersburg PA
CBHW020459030426
42337CB00011B/164